Body, Mind & Food

Wellness Triad through Darwin's Eyes

JONG SOUE YOU, PhD

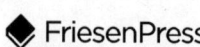 FriesenPress

Suite 300 - 990 Fort St
Victoria, BC, Canada, V8V 3K2
www.friesenpress.com

Copyright © 2015 by Jong Soue You, PhD
First Edition — 2015

All rights reserved.

No part of this publication may be reproduced in any form, or by any means, electronic or mechanical, including photocopying, recording, or any information browsing, storage, or retrieval system, without permission in writing from FriesenPress.

ISBN
978-1-4602-7274-9 (Hardcover)
978-1-4602-7275-6 (Paperback)
978-1-4602-7276-3 (eBook)

1. Health & Fitness

Distributed to the trade by The Ingram Book Company

*Dedicated to
Kathy
and
all women and men, young and old,
with a strong desire to achieve and maintain
a healthy and vibrant
lifestyle.*

Disclaimer

THE AUTHOR'S OPINIONS, IDEAS AND SUGGESTIONS contained in this book are not intended as rendering of medical, health or any other kind of personal professional services. They are intended as helpful and informative material on the subjects discussed in the book. As such, the author specifically disclaims all responsibility for any liability, loss or risk, which may be incurred as a consequence, directly or indirectly, of the use and application of any of the contents of this book.

Dr. Jong Soue You, a retired economics professor, is an economic columnist, bank director, financial planner, and registered retirement consultant (RRC®). As a onetime aspiring scientist, he is an avid reader of scientific literature ranging from Richard Dawkins to Brian Greene. Through integration and synthesis of the body of established wisdom, accumulated scientific knowledge, and his life-long personal experience, Dr. You has distilled seven principles for healthy living. These seven principles are grounded in the Darwinian notion of survival of the fittest, or natural selection of the one most responsive to change. The seven principles are based on the modern theories of biochemistry and human physiology and supported by the solid scientific evidence accumulated to date. The seven principles form a package of natural laws one must obey to achieve and maintain optimum physical, emotional, and mental fitness. Adherence to the seven principles leads to what is known as wellness-triad equilibrium.

This writing was motivated by his strong desire to share the seven principles with a wider community of interested people, particularly all women and men, young and old, with a strong desire to achieve and maintain a healthy and vibrant lifestyle.

Acknowledgements

I AM DEEPLY INDEBTED TO MANY INDIVIDUALS WHO have generously donated their valuable time by reading and critiquing my manuscript and making helpful suggestions. I am particularly indebted to Dr. Eunyong Chung, former Nutrition Advisor to the U.S. Agency for International Development, and to Dr. John J. You, Associate Professor of Medicine, and of Clinical Epidemiology and Biostatistics at McMaster University, for their critical and helpful comments.

My particular thanks go to Dr. Richard Wilson, Distinguished Professor Emeritus at Rutgers University, author and poet, and to Carolyn You, poet and writer, who combed through my manuscript and made helpful comments. I am also thankful to many others who have read and commented on my manuscript at various stages in its progression.

Special thanks are due to my wife, Kathy, former Medical Librarian at Sault Area Hospital, for encouraging me to write and for prodding me to use plain language as much as possible to make this work accessible to a wider audience. I thank the anonymous editor of Friesen Press for helpful and encouraging comments on my manuscript.

I have benefited from the body of accumulated scientific knowledge, particularly in biochemistry, human physiology, genetics, and evolution, as it relates to human diet and physical and mental health. Specifically, I have benefited enormously from various video lectures and courses made available through LearnersTV on the subjects including human physiology; fundamentals of biochemistry & genetics; cell structure & function, genetics & animal development; evolution, ecology & behaviour; Darwin's legacy; eukaryotic gene expression; and essentials of immunology. These courses were lectured by Professors S. Dasgupta (IIT), Robert A. Weinberg/Eric Lander (MIT), Jennifer A. Doudna /Gary L. Firestone/ Michael Meighan/Jasper D. Rine (UC-Irvine), Stephen C. Steams (Yale), William Durham/Robert Siegel/Lynn Rothschild (Stanford), P. N. Rangarajan (IISc), and R. Manjunath (IISc) respectively. For recent scientific evidence on the health effects of diet, physical exercise, and lifestyle stress, I have benefited from the research findings reported in reputable online sources including cancer.gov, diabetes.org, diabetes.ca, diabetes.co.uk, drbenkim.com, en.wikipedia.org, health.gov.on.ca, heart.org, mhp.gov. on.ca, nature.com, ncbi.nlm.gov, nhlbi.nih.gov, nihseniorhealth.gov, nlm.nih.gov, rice.edu, sciencenews.org, and webmd.com. Needless to say, none of the sources mentioned above should bear responsibilities for any errors of commission or omission there may exist in this volume, for which I am solely responsible.

Jong Soue You

Richmond Hill, Ontario, Canada

May, 2015

Table of Contents

Disclaimer v

Acknowledgements vii

Foreword xv

I. Introduction 1

II. Let Nature Take Its Own Course 11

III. Healthy Living:
Sacred Responsibility and Moral Obligation 21

IV. The Nature Of Life On Earth 27

V. Abrupt And Massive Environmental Shocks And Their Effects On Human Health: Physiological Rationale And Supporting Evidence 31

    A. Abrupt and Massive Shocks to the Diet 32

        (I) Blood-Cholesterol-Related Rationale and Evidence 32

        (II) Insulin-Resistance-Related Rationale and Evidence 37

        (III) Oxidative-Stress-Related Rationale and Evidence 39

        (IV) Blood pH-Related Rationale and Evidence 44

        (V) Health Effects of Abrupt and Massive Shocks to the Way Food is Grown, Raised, Processed, and Prepared 46

B. Abrupt and Massive Shocks to the Level of Physical Activity..50

C. Abrupt and Massive Shocks to the State of Mind.....52

VI. Seven Principles For Healthy Living............................55

Principle 1. Healthy Living Starts With Working Towards A Healthy Body And Mind..57

Principle 2. A Healthy Body And Mind Is Achieved Through A Healthy, Balanced Diet, An Appropriate Amount Of Physical Exercise, And Maintaining A Peaceful And Cheerful Mind. 60

Principle 3. A Healthy, Balanced Diet Is Best Achieved Through The Intake Of A Variety Of Foods From A Variety Of Sources, Preferably Plant And Marine-Life Based, In As Natural A State As Possible.......................63

Principle 4: How Much One Eats Is Not As Critical For Human Health As What One Eats. 75

Principle 5: The Appropriate Amount Of Physical Exercise Depends On One's Age And The Existing Level Of Physical Fitness. 77

Principle 6: A Peaceful And Cheerful Mind Is Attained Through Self-Respect, Respect For Others, Respect For Nature, A Positive Attitude Toward Life, And Occasional Quiet Moments...82

Principle 7: The Ideal Body Weight Is The One Associated With One's Optimum Physical And Mental Fitness, Not A Specific Number On A Scale. 85

VII. Putting The Seven Principles Into Practice 87

A. How To Achieve And Maintain A Properly Balanced, Healthy Diet 88

 B. Some Observations on Species Diets and their Longevity 106

 C. Achieving And Maintaining Physical Fitness 110

 D. Disciplining Of The Mind 118

VIII. Closing Words 125

A Mathematical Appendix 133

Index 137

Organizing our thoughts on healthy living within the context of the Darwinian theory of evolution may itself be a revolutionary idea.

Foreword

ANYONE WALKING INTO A BOOKSTORE WILL FIND numerous books on the subject of health and wellness. Why then another book on the subject? Why a book on health and wellness written by a non-expert (or a "deemed" non-expert) on the subject? There are at least two reasons that justify my writing on the subject: The first and foremost reason is that, despite the great number of books on the subject inundating the market, the lifestyle of the human species is not becoming healthier, and if anything, is becoming less healthy day by day, even as I write this book. To prove this point, we only need to be reminded of the obesity epidemic, which the World Health Organization has identified as one of the most serious non-communicable health risks threatening the world's population and currently the most significant contributor to premature human mortality. The second reason, which may not be obvious to readers, but I hope will become more persuasive in the following pages, is this: Experts in the health professions have failed in persuading and convincing the general population that human lifestyle must change drastically and without delay if a major calamity is to be avoided. This could be due to the unfortunate fact that the perspectives of the experts are not broad and far sighted enough to allow them to see the true nature of the problem clearly. To put it differently, it may be their restricted frame of reference, with its extremely narrow focus (which their chosen disciplines tend to require), that is the root of the problem. Sometimes it takes stepping back and a fresh perspective, with a different frame of reference that only outsiders or non-experts can provide, to make the core of the problem more clearly visible.

After all, it is not the paucity of information and knowledge that is the problem. Rather it is the lack of a fresh perspective and sense of urgency that seems to be the real problem. As a non-expert who has struggled for many decades to gain a better understanding of human health and wellness issues, I propose in this book a fresh perspective: that healthy living can only be attained and maintained by living in harmony with nature. Living in harmony with nature means that our body and mind are allowed to adjust naturally to the constantly changing life environment, in accordance with the natural process of human evolutionary adaptation, and that our body and mind are not subjected to excessive amounts and frequencies of harmful external, particularly man-made, shocks as much as possible. External man-made shocks that are harmful to our body and mind are the abrupt and massive shocks that are being generated externally as a result (mainly) of the rapid industrialization and technological change that has taken place in an extremely short span of time – too short for the human body and mind, with limited inherent genetic abilities, to respond to adequately. These swift and massive environmental changes have had far-reaching negative consequences on our lifestyle, ranging from the unhealthy foods we eat to the inappropriate level of physical activity to work environments that induce emotional and mental stress.

In this book, I present seven principles for healthy living. The seven principles are grounded in the Darwinian notion of survival of the fittest, or natural selection of the one most responsive to change – the one best capable of adapting to a changing life environment. The seven principles are based on the modern theories of biochemistry and human physiology, and strongly supported by the body of scientific evidence accumulated to date. In this sense, they form a package of natural laws one must obey to achieve and maintain an optimum physical, emotional, and mental fitness. The driving force behind the seven principles is the perspective of Darwinian natural selection. The seven principles lead to a triad of essential requirements for healthy living: a healthy, balanced diet, an appropriate level of physical activity, and a harmonious state of mind. This notion of triad is not new. What is new is the theoretical framework and perspective that is used to develop the proposition, and the way in which the scientific evidence is organized and presented to support and operationalize the proposition.

This writing is motivated by my strong desire to share the seven principles for healthy living with a wider community of interested people, particularly all women and men with a strong desire to achieve and maintain a healthy and vibrant lifestyle. The book presents practical and concrete steps for achieving the triad of essential requirements for healthy living and for maintaining the triad in a state of stable equilibrium. These steps are specifically designed to respect the natural process of human evolutionary adaptation and the principle of living in harmony with nature. The book is designed as a lifetime companion, a reference book for all women and men, young and old, who strongly desire to achieve and maintain a healthy body and mind. It is hoped that as many people as possible will come to read this book. The book also provides a philosophical basis for healthy living and the pursuit of happiness as individual's sacred responsibility and moral obligation.

I. Introduction

"If you held hands with your mother, and she held hands with hers, and she with hers, the line would stretch only from New York to Washington before you were holding hands with the "missing link" – the common ancestor with chimpanzees."

~ Matt Ridley

ALL THINGS IN THE UNIVERSE ARE THE OUTCOMES OF the evolutionary process. They are, in fact, products in process, rather than finished products. Some, like human beings, are organic in nature. Others, like rocks, are inorganic. Whether organic or inorganic, they all share a common ancestor or origin: matters that constitute the universe and a set of fundamental forces governing the movement and evolution of the universe and its constituent parts, ranging in size from sub-atomic elementary particles to planets, stars, and galaxies. Modern science has identified four fundamental forces of nature governing the movement and evolution of the universe and its constituent parts. They are as follows: the gravitational force, the electromagnetic force, the strong nuclear force, and the weak nuclear force. Albert Einstein felt that the four fundamental forces may be four different manifestations of a single even more fundamental force yet to be identified.

The human body, like all other things in the universe, is governed by the four fundamental forces (or a single even more fundamental force of nature yet to be identified). As such, the way the human body functions, like the way all other things in the universe behave, obeys the basic laws of physics and chemistry. Understanding of human wellness or disorder must start from this premise. The human body, like all things in the universe, is an evolutionary product in process.

What is evolution? Evolution is a process of adaptation by an entity, organic or inorganic, to a changing environment within the constraints of the fundamental forces of nature. Charles Darwin, one of the greatest human thinkers who ever lived (referring obviously to the evolution of organic life forms), stated: "It is not the strongest of the species that survives, nor the most intelligent, but the one most responsive to change." Alfred Russell Wallace and other thinkers contemporary to Darwin had basically the same idea, but it was Darwin who painstakingly amassed a wealth of evidence, organized it for over twenty years, and publicly presented his idea in a monumental volume, *On the Origin of Species*, in 1859. Evolution is value-neutral. It is neither progression nor regression. It is just a process of adaptation to a changing environment. Hence it cannot be argued that human beings are more or less advanced evolutionarily than hummingbirds, or yeast bacteria. They have just evolved in different directions through adaptation to changes in their respective environments. Human beings may be the most intelligent but not necessarily the most advanced from the evolutionary point of view. One of many misconceptions about evolution frequently encountered is that the human species has evolved from the primates like monkeys or chimpanzees. This is, of course, not the case. What is true is that all primates, including the human species, have evolved from their common ancestor in different directions, through adaptation to changes in their respective environments. In fact, the theory of evolution says that all life forms have evolved from their common ancestor – the first living organism to appear on earth – all in different directions. Along the way, further successive branching out (in different directions) has occurred from the successive common ancestors. What is absolutely true is that all living organisms face the same destiny: adjust or perish.

How and why did organic life forms evolve from inorganic matter? One can imagine that, when the matters reconfigure themselves, they attempt to do this in the most efficient or economical way possible, within the constraints of the four fundamental forces of nature. They must solve an economic problem of constrained optimization every time they reconfigure themselves physically or chemically. For example, light travels in a straight line to minimize the cost in terms of time and effort (energy), within the constraints of the gravitational and other fundamental forces acting upon it. Why are snowflakes perfectly symmetrical in shape? It could be that the symmetrical shape is the most efficient or economical shape to sustain. Why are crystals perfectly symmetrical in shape? Presumably for the same reason that the snowflakes have a symmetrical shape. In fact, the crystals that grow may be regarded as the harbinger of organic life forms, since what distinguishes the organic from the inorganic is the ability of the former to grow and multiply itself. It stands to reason that, in a primeval soup of extreme temperature and extreme pressure, the matters attempting to reconfigure themselves within the constraints of the fundamental forces of nature in the most efficient or economical way, i.e., by obeying the law of symmetry among others, may have hit upon a secret that produced the first living organism by pure accident ... or perhaps this was inevitable. In fact, it is believed that life on earth appeared rather soon after the birth of the planet earth about 4.5 billion years ago – almost as soon as the surface of the earth cooled enough to form water, about 3.6 - 3.9 billion years ago – even with little or no oxygen. This suggests that the emergence of life on earth was an inevitable natural phenomenon rather than a low-probability chance occurrence. The emergence of the first living organism would have triggered the inevitable process of the evolution of organic life forms. The process of evolution, however, was extremely slow initially. The very early life forms were in fact pre-cellular RNAs (ribonucleic acids), units of genetic material. When the first prokaryotic cells evolved from the pre-cellular life forms, they didn't yet have nucleus in them (e.g., bacteria and archaea). It took prokaryotic cells some 2 billion years to develop nucleus and evolve into eukaryotic cells, which were still unicellular (e.g., amoeba). It took another billion years for these unicellular organisms to evolve into multicellular organisms. Presumably the extremely slow process of evolution was due to the lack of oxygen. Until about 600 million years ago, when the green plants and algae started releasing oxygen into the biosphere as a by-product of photosynthesis, there was little oxygen in the environment. Once oxygen became abundantly available, multicellular organisms proliferated quickly and the evolution of life acquired a great momentum. The plants and animals emerged within 50 million years after that. Higher forms of life evolved only because of the presence of oxygen, which made it possible for the organisms to generate more energy. The human species appeared quite recently, only about 150 - 200 thousand years ago. Chimpanzees, our closest living relative, branched out from our common ancestor family about 4 - 6 million years ago. In the long process of evolution, many new life forms emerged and many existing life forms became extinct. Those that could not adjust perished.

The Darwinian theory of evolution is applicable not only to the evolution of organic species on planet earth but to the evolution of the universe itself (Richard Dawkins, *The Blind Watchmaker*, 1986). It is a powerful theory capable of explaining a wide range of phenomena in the universe. A growing body of scientific evidence seems to suggest that the insights from this theory are applicable to an inquiry into the nature and causes of the sickness and health of the human body and mind. It may not be an exaggeration to suggest that the problem of human wellness can best be understood within the broad context of the Darwinian theory of evolution.

What kinds of food should we eat and how much? What levels of physical activity should we aim for? What state of mind should we strive to attain and maintain, for wellbeing of our body and mind? These questions can best be understood and answered within the broad context of the Darwinian theory of natural selection or survival of the fittest. Scientific evidence for this proposition is clear, abundant, persuasive, and in fact, rock-solid in my view. And yet we do not see it. Perhaps we choose to ignore it, because we do not have the courage to admit and face it. Or worse still, perhaps we are so deeply immersed in our present deceptive culture, and the routine of our day-to-day living, that we are incapable of seeing the truth through the fog of confusion and the maze of unorganized knowledge and information. Or perhaps the truth is so tantalizingly simple that we do not recognize it even when it is left bare right before our eyes. But then, aren't all truths simple?

The magnitude, seriousness, and urgency of the health problem facing us as humans today, both physical and mental, are vastly greater than we choose to admit. The lifestyles we cling to determine the kinds of food we eat, the levels of physical activity we undertake, and the state of mind we are in. They are only the immediate causes of the problem. The root cause of the problem, however, lies in our inability to see what has brought about these immediate causes. We are blind to the fact that it is predominantly the rapidly accelerating pace of change in our life environment, chiefly attributable to ever-intensifying industrialization and technological change (to which human physiology has great difficulty adjusting), that is the root cause of the problem. Our life environment is changing much too fast for our body and mind to adjust to it. Our thirst for the accelerating pace of technological change seems to be unquenchable. The human physiological-response rate to the accelerating man-made changes in the human life environment, at the present stage of human evolution, appears much too inadequate for the species' health or perhaps even survival. Our only practical option to achieve individual survival in the short run, short of slowing down the pace of change in our external environment, is to deliberately counteract these forces as much as possible at the individual level. This is what I propose in this book. I leave the greater task of dealing with the pace of man-made environmental change itself to the experts in the field.

Sceptics may ask, "Isn't evolutionary time scale too enormous to apply it to what appears to be rather short-run issues of human health and wellness? What must be remembered, however, is the fact that what has taken millions or billions of years to evolve can be wiped out literally overnight by an abrupt and massive environmental shock. What has happened to the human life environment in the last centuries (and even decades) in the industrialized world is nothing short of an abrupt and massive shock. Compare the foods we eat today to what our parents used to eat. In fact, what some of us ourselves eat now compared to what we used to eat only decades ago! Take a note of the extent to which food is now grown, raised, refined, processed, prepared and cooked compared to earlier times. The same goes for the level of physical inactivity and lifestyle stress. Think about, for instance, our near total dependence on automobiles, electronic gadgets, and such in our daily lives of today. Nothing short of abrupt and massive environmental shock indeed!

The seven principles presented here are rooted in the notion that all organic life forms have acquired, through the course of evolution, an inherent genetic ability to adapt to changes in their life environment and to neutralize adverse external shocks; however, the faster the pace of change in their life environment, and the greater the frequency and intensity of the adverse external shocks to which the life forms are subjected, the more compromised their ability to cope with and survive these shocks will be. Some primitive organisms, like antibiotics-resistant bacteria, seem to adapt quite well and fairly quickly to the changes in their life environment. Highly complex organisms like dinosaurs, on the other hand, failed miserably to adapt to sudden and massive adverse external shocks and couldn't escape extinction. It is not at all clear whether the human species will be able to overcome or adapt successfully to the current wave of sudden and intensive adverse external shocks that are being incessantly hurled against them. What is clear is that necessary corrective measures are urgently needed both at the individual and societal levels if the human species is to avoid a major calamity or even a biological extinction.

In the modern industrial and information age in which we humans live, the frequency and intensity of man-made adverse shocks are making our life environment less and less hospitable. Our way of life, including what we do, what we eat, what we drink, how we play, and what and how we think and feel, is moving further and further away from what would have been the case had the gradual process of human evolutionary adaptation been allowed to take its own natural course without massive human intervention. In order not to be swept away by this torrential current of "unnatural" lifestyle, one must be vigilant in resisting it. Any approach to healthy living that does not respect the natural process of gradual human evolutionary adaptation is bound to fail. There is a danger that hastily drawn-up prescriptions for healthy living, without due regard to the principle of living in harmony with nature, may be counterproductive. More will be said about this later.

Readers will find that some widely held beliefs based on conventional wisdom about healthy living are false, while some others are supported by common sense, everyday life experience, and scientific evidence. Conventional wisdom often tends to emphasize getting results through man-made corrective measures, be it forced diet plans or an unnatural exercise regimen. Our bodies should not be subjected to artificial or unnatural shocks except in medical emergencies. Our bodies have evolved, through the process of natural selection, to function best when allowed to work in harmony with nature, respecting the natural process of human evolutionary adaptation. Any reasonable approach to achieving and maintaining a healthy lifestyle must respect this evolutionary fact.

Could it be that organizing our thoughts on healthy living in the context of the theory of evolution is itself a revolutionary idea?

II. Let Nature Take Its Own Course

"It is not the strongest of the species that survives, nor the most intelligent, but the one most responsive to change."

~ *Charles Darwin*

BY AND LARGE, THE NATURAL ENVIRONMENT OF planet earth undergoes gradual, with intermittently violent, changes by an evolutionary standard within the evolving universe. Organic species on earth try to adapt to this changing environment in order to survive and prosper. Over the course of the long period of natural selection, all organic species have developed self-defence mechanisms or immune systems to fight off or neutralize external shocks that are harmful to their bodies and that threaten their survival. All organisms are constantly exposed to compounds that they cannot use as foods and would be harmful if accumulated in cells. These xenobiotics are detoxified by a set of xenobiotic-metabolizing enzymes, for example, lysozymes, within our body. Invading pathogens are attacked and killed by antibodies produced by the body's immune system. All organisms must maintain a set of constant conditions within cells, a healthy condition known as homeostasis, to stay healthy. This remarkable self-defence mechanism, however, has its limitations. When subjected to harmful external shocks long enough, or when shocks are abrupt and strong enough, the defensive mechanism crumbles and the body either contracts diseases or its health gradually or suddenly deteriorates. These harmful external shocks come in the form of the polluted air we breathe, the polluted water we drink, and the unhealthy or contaminated foods we eat (unhealthy from a dietary point of view, contaminated with preservatives and pesticides, or refined and processed to such an extent as to weaken and damage the body's digestive, absorptive, circulatory, and waste removal functions). When harmful external shocks come gradually in small dosages, the self-defence mechanism may not have difficulty handling them. When they come suddenly in great quantities and frequencies, however, it may be too much for the mechanism to cope with. This is because the body is not allowed to take a natural course of gradual evolutionary adaptation but is instead subjected to a sudden and intensive bombardment of harmful external shocks, frequently man-made.

Body, Mind & Food

The foods that the human species eats have evolved over billions of years through the evolutionary process from the time of simple non-cellular organic molecule to the present day diet for the complex multi-cellular organism. Considering the stages of evolution the human species has traversed for the last 150 to 200 thousand years, it is highly likely that the diet of the early ancestors of the human species must have consisted mainly of plant-based foods. Only recently (perhaps within less than a hundred thousand years), the diet for the humans must have been expanded to include some animal-based foods, necessitated by the sheer need to satisfy their hunger, even though their diet to this day is still primarily plant based. The discovery of fire, and of cooking by fire, would have allowed the human diet to progress further and faster to one that is more animal based. The natural and healthy human diet, however, remains primarily plant based even to this day. Professor Nathaniel Dominy, a pioneer in the field of human diet evolution, presents the most compelling evidence for this. According to Dominy, anatomically humans are not adapted to an animal-based diet at all; for example, the shape and alignment of human teeth are not suited for an animal-based diet. Dominy presents strong evidence that a major driving force behind the hominid bipedalism, and the gradual increase in human brain size, has been the mix of plant foods with a large amount of starch coming from tubers and seeds, which has been for a long time (and still) is the fundamental component of the human diet. The fact that the diet of chimpanzees, our closest evolutionary cousin, is mostly fruit and vegetation corroborates this line of reasoning. Dominy's findings are not surprising considering the obvious likelihood that, along the evolutionary paths, the diet of our human ancestors (simple organisms initially) must have started with what was available at the time in the organic world, and must have expanded gradually to include newly emerging species. That inclusion of newly emerging species in the normal diet must have required lengthy periods of physiological adaptation. This line of reasoning naturally leads to a proposition that the greater a food source's evolutionary (genetic) distance is from the human species the more natural a component of human diet it is, and thus the more beneficial for human health it is likely to be. To put it differently, the smaller a food source's evolutionary distance is from the human species, the more unnatural a component of human diet it is and thus the less beneficial for human health it is likely to be. While all life on earth shares a common ancestor, evolution has produced (over billions of years) a vast array of species, branching out in all directions. Of this infinitely large number of species, some are healthier than others as a human dietary source, depending on their evolutionary distance from humans. In terms of healthiness as a human dietary source, we recognize, for instance, that avocado is farther distanced from the human species evolutionarily than is chicken, and hence avocado is healthier than chicken as a source of fat for humans to consume. Similarly, the evolutionary distance between chickens and humans is greater than that between cows and humans, which implies that chicken fat is healthier than beef fat for humans to consume. Incidentally, this logic would compel us to repudiate cannibalism on the basis of health reasons quite independently of moral grounds. Here, without going into the full detail of the evolutionary tree and broadly speaking, we merely point out the fact that plant species are farther distanced evolutionarily from the human species than are animal species and that, within the class of animal species, the respective evolutionary distance from the human species of fish, amphibians, birds, and mammals decreases progressively in that order.

This logic naturally implies that a predominantly plant-based diet is healthier for humans than a diet that is predominantly animal based. The fact that humans cannot survive on an entirely animal-based diet for very long (for example, scurvy) but can survive and even prosper on an entirely plant-based diet lends additional support to the proposition. This suggests that until human physiology is well adapted to animal-based diet through further evolutionary adaptation, which could be many millennia away or quite likely even longer, animal-based foods may not be as healthy for humans as plant-based foods and should only be taken in moderation. The process of evolutionary adaptation for complex organisms such as humans is quite slow. Needless to say, the proposition does not condemn all animal-based foods as equally unhealthy, but states that healthiness of a food source depends on its evolutionary distance from the human species. Thus, even within the class of animal-based foods the evolutionary distance from the human species is a critical factor in determining how beneficial a particular food source is to human health. A food source's evolutionary distance from the human species can be regarded as a proxy for the measure of human physiological adaptation to the particular food source.

Until recently, humans had no shortage of the physical labour required for survival. With the passing of the agrarian society, and the advent of the industrial age (and now the information age), came less and less need for physical labour and more and more need for office-related work skills. For the first time in human history, an insufficient amount of physical activity has become a health concern, as a result of the abrupt man-made departure from the natural course of gradual evolutionary adaptation. This unnatural living condition, if left uncorrected, will spell disaster for the human species. We must raise the level of human physical activity to what is more in sync with the natural course of gradual, human-evolutionary adaptation.

Admittedly human life expectancy has dramatically improved since the industrial revolution, while the level of human physical activity has actually decreased, and the human diet has become more animal based. One may ask: Doesn't this imply that the decreased level of physical activity and a diet that is more animal based are responsible for the improved life expectancy of the human species? This may be true to a certain extent. The abject poverty that prevailed during the pre-industrial age deprived the masses of a nutritious diet. This combined with back-breaking labour may have contributed to early death. A primitive state of medicine that was unable to cope with even common infectious diseases and poor hygiene must have exacerbated the situation. However, while it could be said that vastly improved economic conditions in the industrial and information age, combined with the advancement of modern medicine, have certainly eliminated hunger in the developed world and have raised human life expectancy to an unprecedented level, it cannot be denied that there is a mountain of evidence that a lack of sufficient physical activity coupled with a diet rich in animal fat and highly refined carbohydrates and sugar are contributing to the early deaths of many people who would live much longer, in better health, free from a constant and losing battle to shed pounds. The pendulum has swung in a short span of time from one extreme of hunger and back-breaking labour to the other extreme of over-eating and insufficient physical activity. This seems to suggest that the maximum human life expectancy associated with healthy diet and healthy lifestyle could be significantly greater than what it is today. In fact, evidence is clearly pointing in that direction, as we will see in later chapters.

With the faster and faster pace of life brought about by the industrial and information age, another sign of abrupt departure from the gradual change in natural human environment, it has become critically important and yet increasingly difficult for humans to be close to nature and to maintain a peaceful and cheerful mind. Going back to nature would greatly help us restore peaceful and cheerful minds. When this is not practically feasible, distancing ourselves occasionally (on a daily basis) from a hectic pace of life, through such simple mind-control exercises as deep breathing and positive thinking, could go a long way in helping us restore peaceful and cheerful minds. On a more fundamental level, it can be argued that self-respect, respect for others, respect for nature, a positive attitude toward life, and occasional quiet moments are the key minimum ingredients for the attainment of a peaceful and cheerful mind. Further discussion on this will follow.

It is well worth remembering Charles Darwin's penetrating insight: "It is not the strongest of the species that survives, nor the most intelligent, but the one most responsive to change." We humans may be the most intelligent of the species ever to have lived on planet earth. Are we the most responsive to change as well? Or are we short-sighted and foolish enough to have caused the most massive and disruptive change to our life environment that ever occurred in the history of the human species, to which we may not be able to successfully adapt? It is perhaps time to sound an alarm bell and re-examine our lifestyle thoroughly. It is perhaps time to reorient our lifestyle, before it is too late, and start living in harmony with nature. Living in harmony with nature means respecting the natural process of human evolutionary adaptation in what we eat and drink, in how we work and play, and in what and how we think and feel.

III. Healthy Living: Sacred Responsibility and Moral Obligation

> "*Know ye not that ye are the temple of God, and [that] the Spirit of God dwelleth in you?*"
>
> ~ *1 Corinthians 3:16-17*

IF THERE IS A COMMON DENOMINATOR FOR ALL RELIgions, it must be the belief that God created the world. The world here is to be interpreted as the entire universe, including all life forms within it. A corollary to this statement is that when God created life forms, He must have intended for them to live. "To live," of course, means "to live, prosper and propagate." It must then follow that any act harming the lives of living creatures, including human beings and the environment in which we live, is against the will of God. Further, it must then be recognized that it is a sacred responsibility and moral obligation of all living creatures, including human beings, to look after their bodies and minds to the best of their abilities to ensure healthy living, both as an individual and as a member of the community. This responsibility and obligation of course extends to the environment in which all life forms live. This line of reasoning also suggests that it is a serious crime to harm not only your own body and mind but that of your fellow living creatures, and further that there is no bigger crime in the eyes of God than harming one's own body or mind.

It is said that "You are the temple of God" or "God dwells within you." These statements may be interpreted as meaning that God, as the Creator, cares for you and watches you every step of the way after you are born and does not abandon you once you are cast into the world. You have a responsibility and obligation to keep your body and mind clean and healthy, suitable as God's dwelling. Neglecting this responsibility and obligation is a serious crime. Along with this responsibility and obligation comes our duty to respect the same responsibility and obligation of fellow living creatures, including fellow human beings as God's creations.

As for the minds of other creatures, there seems to be a presumption, widely shared by humans (human chauvinists?), that consciousness and emotional capacity are faculties unique to the human species. Scientific evidence clearly contradicts this misconception. It is now well-known that a variety of animals are capable of showing a wide range of emotions and various levels of intelligence. Animals that show sadness and feelings of hurt by crying tears include chimpanzees, gorillas, orangutans, whales, elephants, dugongs (sea cows), cows, horses, donkeys, and camels. Animals show their capacity for thoughts and emotions in a variety of ways. I have personally witnessed numerous occasions of my Havanese puppy being immersed in what can only be described as deep thinking. I have observed a gorilla in the Metropolitan Toronto Zoo clearly in deep thought. It was a sunny summer afternoon. She was sitting with her chin propped up by one of her palms, blinking her eyes as if trying to figure something out, scratching her head as if in puzzlement and twiddling the index finger of her other free hand on the ground, as if trying to concentrate or focus her mind on something. Professor Marc Bekoff, who has studied animal emotions for thirty years (*The Emotional Lives of Animals*, 2007), confirms that mammals, birds, and fish experience rich and deep emotional lives, feeling passions from pure and contagious joy during play to deep grief and pain.

Morals governing our relationship with non-human creatures may be more complex and uncertain than those governing human to human relationships, but there is little doubt that they should be based on the same fundamental principle. According to this principle, it may be said that harming one's body or mind is the most serious crime (affront to divine intention), harming the bodies and minds of fellow human beings is the second most serious crime, harming the bodies and minds of fellow non-human living creatures is the third most serious crime, harming the environment in which we all live is the fourth most serious crime, and so forth. This ordering is only illustrative and no doubt reflects my subjective human point of view. In any case, it seems clear that we have a sacred responsibility and moral obligation to look after our own bodies and minds to the best of our ability, to ensure our physical, emotional, and mental health. We do not have a right to abuse or harm our own body or mind. This has to be true regardless of one's religious orientation. As God's creations, we must respect ourselves, other living organisms (including fellow human beings), and the environment in which we all live. Only then will we be able to achieve a peaceful and cheerful mind in harmony with nature.

Along with the right to live comes the right to pursue happiness – pursuit of happiness being one of the fundamental instincts of life. The right to pursue happiness includes the right to pursue secular pleasures. It goes without saying, however, that pursuit of secular pleasures must be restrained by the consideration that the acts of pursuing these pleasures should not harm your own body and mind or the bodies and minds of fellow human beings and of other living creatures, or the environment in which we all live. Other than that, there should be no constraint placed on an individual's inherent right to pursue happiness, including secular pleasures.

It is God's will that we live healthy. It is God's will that we live in happiness. As God's children then, not only do we have a right to live healthy and in happiness but also we have a sacred responsibility and a moral obligation to live healthy lives in happiness!

IV. The Nature Of Life On Earth

WHAT IS LIFE? LIFE IS A PROCESS OF ADAPTING TO A changing environment, nothing more and nothing less. The purpose of life in a fundamental sense is to live and multiply, and to do this in the most efficient way possible, given environmental constraints. All living organisms must solve a set of fundamental, economic, constrained-optimization problems, on an ongoing basis. Optimization can take the form of maximization of benefits under a given set of cost constraints or minimization of costs under a given set of benefit (budget) constraints. In fact, this is not unique to organic life forms. Rather it is universal in that even inorganic matters must solve a set of constrained-optimization problems (represented by a set of differential equations) in order to comply with the fundamental laws of nature. For example, rays of sunlight must travel in a straight line to minimize time and effort (energy expended) within the constraints of fundamental forces of nature. All laws of nature must reflect the fundamental economic principle of constrained optimization.

This fundamental principle applies to the movements of all matters in the universe, whether constituents of a living organism or inorganic matter, as they reconfigure themselves while travelling along their evolutionary trajectories. All things in the universe, whether organic or inorganic, must obey the fundamental laws of nature and the basic laws of physics and chemistry in particular. This view of the universe does not seem to fundamentally contradict the foundation on which all of the world's religions are based. This is the premise on which our understanding of human wellness should be based.

For organic life forms, solving a set of constrained optimization problems means responding and adapting to a changing life environment as best as possible under the given set of constraints. A good example of this is presented in a recent book by Richard Dawkins (*The Greatest Show on Earth: The Evidence for Evolution*, 2009), which describes how optimum heights of individual trees or various species of trees in a given geographical area are determined by carefully balancing the marginal benefit of additional sunlight that additional height provides, and the marginal cost of additional nutrients (energy) required for the additional height. This process of constrained optimization is continuous and ongoing for all living organisms. In efforts to live and multiply, living organisms continuously respond and adapt to the continuously changing environment through the process of genetic mutations, i.e., the process of evolution. When environmental changes are too abrupt and massive for them to respond successfully, the organisms or species may be forced into extinction. Extinction of species is, of course, not instantaneous. Species are likely to go through various stages of unsuccessful adaptation (health problems) prior to eventual extinction. Simple organisms, such as viruses and bacteria, tend to be more responsive and better able to adapt to environmental changes than are complex organisms such as dinosaurs and humans.

As for the human species in the early twenty-first century, it seems too early to even speculate whether it would be able to adapt successfully to the torrential wave of environmental changes that are currently taking place at an accelerating pace on three different fronts: diet, level of physical activity, and state of mind. At the individual level at least, it would make good sense for everyone to try to minimize, to the extent possible, the effects on the individual that these environmental changes bring about in the three areas of diet, physical activity, and state of mind.

In what follows, we will examine how the human body can be harmed by improper diet, inadequate level of physical activity, and emotional and mental stress, using the knowledge we have gained in human physiology and the supporting scientific evidence we have acquired to date.

V. Abrupt And Massive Environmental Shocks And Their Effects On Human Health: Physiological Rationale And Supporting Evidence

"All the energy that drives life comes ultimately from sunlight trapped by plants."

~ Richard Dawkins

IN THIS CHAPTER, PHYSIOLOGICAL RATIONALE AND supporting scientific evidence for the damaging effects that abrupt and massive environmental shocks (from an evolutionary point of view) have on human health will be examined. Abrupt and massive environmental shocks to humans come in the forms of abrupt and massive shocks to the diet, to the physical activity level, and to the state of mind.

A. Abrupt and Massive Shocks to the Diet

Presentation of the material in this section will be grouped into the following five broad categories:

(I) blood-cholesterol-related rationale and evidence;

(II) insulin-resistance-related rationale and evidence;

(III) oxidative-stress-related rationale and evidence;

(IV) blood pH-related rationale and evidence: and

(V) health effects of abrupt and massive shocks to the way food is grown, raised, processed, and prepared.

(I) Blood-Cholesterol-Related Rationale and Evidence

Cholesterol has a bad reputation. It is, however, a vital compound found in the blood and in every cell of our body. It is a variety of lipid and is one of the essential building blocks of cell membranes. Cholesterol is essential as well for the synthesizing of vitamin D and many hormones. Too much cholesterol in the blood, however, is known to increase the risk of heart disease and stroke, by leading to a buildup of plaque on artery walls. The plaque buildup, if allowed to persist, can narrow the arteries and reduce blood flow. If a blood clot forms, and blocks an artery to the heart, a heart attack can occur. If a blood clot blocks an artery to, or in, the brain, a stroke results. It is thus important to ensure that a proper balance of cholesterol in the blood is maintained. Studies have shown that a healthy, balanced diet, appropriate level of physical exercise, and peaceful and cheerful state of mind can all help ensure a proper balance of cholesterol in the blood.

Distinction should be made between blood cholesterol (cholesterol synthesized in the body) and dietary cholesterol (cholesterol found in foods). It is the blood cholesterol, not dietary cholesterol, which is relevant to the present discussion. Dietary cholesterol does not necessarily translate into blood cholesterol. Cholesterol is transported in the blood by lipoproteins. There are two main types of cholesterol:

a. Low-density lipoproteins (LDLs) deliver cholesterol to the cell membrane LDL receptors. This type is often called "bad" cholesterol because too much LDL cholesterol, relative to what the membrane receptors are prepared to accept, can build up on artery walls.

b. High-density lipoproteins (HDLs) remove LDL cholesterol from artery walls and carry it back to the liver. For this reason, HDL cholesterol is called "good" cholesterol.

Blood cholesterol levels are closely linked to intake of dietary fat. It has been found that the foods that raise LDL blood cholesterol the most are saturated fat and trans fat. Saturated fats are found in foods such as fatty meats, full-fat milk products, butter, lard, and those made with hydrogenated vegetable oil. Trans fats are found mainly in foods made with shortening or partially hydrogenated vegetable oil. Most fast foods and snack foods, and many prepared foods, tend to be rich in both saturated fats and trans fats. Trans fats are believed to be the worst kind, because they not only raise LDL cholesterol but also lower HDL cholesterol. On the other hand, foods that contain unsaturated fats (mono or polyunsaturated fats) tend to lower LDL cholesterol and raise HDL cholesterol in the blood. Mono-unsaturated fats are found in avocados, nuts and seeds, and vegetable oils. (Mono-unsaturated fats are liquid at room temperature but harden in the refrigerator.) Polyunsaturated fats are found in fatty fish oils (especially, in mackerel, lake trout, herring, sardines, albacore tuna, and salmon), nuts and seeds, and vegetable oils. (Polyunsaturated fats remain liquid even at colder temperatures.) Nuts, seeds, and vegetable oils contain both mono- and polyunsaturated fats. Most vegetables and fruits also lower LDL cholesterol in the blood. Soluble fibre, found in foods such as oatmeal, kidney beans, Brussel sprouts, apples, pears, psyllium, barley, and prunes tend to lower LDL cholesterol as well.

A closer look at these lists suggests that diets consisting of vegetables, fruits, nuts, and fatty fish contribute to the lowering of LDL cholesterol and the raising of HDL cholesterol in the blood, whereas diets consisting of fatty meats, dairy products, and fast foods have the opposite effects. This seems to suggest that the further removed a food source is from the human species in terms of evolutionary distance, the healthier it is for humans, as far as its impact on the blood cholesterol is concerned. Vegetables, fruits, nuts, and fish are all at a greater distance evolutionarily from the human species than are the animals whose fatty meat and dairy products contribute to high LDL cholesterol levels.

There is no direct correlation between the intake of dietary cholesterol and the blood cholesterol level. Studies have shown that some foods high in cholesterol, such as eggs, shrimps, and scallops do not raise LDL cholesterol in the blood. It is the intake of saturated fats that is responsible for raising the blood LDL cholesterol, not necessarily the intake of foods high in cholesterol. It has been found that fats contained in chicken eggs, shrimps, and scallops are mostly unsaturated fats. For example, more than 70 percent of the fat contained in chicken eggs is unsaturated fat. Studies have also found that these cholesterol rich foods increase the size of LDL particles, making them less likely to stick to artery walls. Specifically, eating sea foods rich in dietary cholesterol, such as shrimps and scallops, does not increase but in fact reduce the risk of cardiovascular disease and stroke. Both kinds of seafood have overwhelmingly more unsaturated fat than saturated fat, and relatively low amounts of both. Needless to say, for this to be the case, they would have to be cooked without sauces or other ingredients that themselves contain high amounts of saturated fats.

Coconut oil is known to be high in saturated fat, but its fat is made up of a unique blend of medium-chain fatty acids. Animal fats are long-chain fatty acids. Unlike long-chain fats, medium-chain ones do not have to be broken down in the small intestine. Because they are smaller, they're absorbed intact and delivered directly to the liver. Studies have found that diets high in coconut oil do raise total blood cholesterol but raise HDL cholesterol more than they do LDL cholesterol, with a net beneficial effect. Coconut oil has been found to facilitate calorie burning in the body as well. Coconut oil also has a high smoke point, which makes it suited for high-heat cooking, with reduced risk of the oxidative stress commonly associated with high-heat cooking in oil (see subsection (III) below for discussion on oxidative stress).

These findings indicate that the plant foods and sea foods and even eggs that are high in cholesterol content do not raise the blood LDL cholesterol and do not increase the risk of heart disease or stroke, unlike the saturated fats contained in the other animal foods. These findings thus lend strong support to the proposition that the greater a food source's evolutionary distance is from the human species, the healthier it is for humans. The plant-based foods, like coconut oil, sea foods like shrimps and scallops, and chicken eggs are all farther away evolutionarily from the human species than are other saturated fat-rich animals. In terms of degree of healthiness, coconut oil would rank the first, shrimps and scallops next, followed by eggs next, and mammals last.

(II) Insulin-Resistance-Related Rationale and Evidence

During digestion and absorption, the carbohydrates in the food we eat are broken down into their simplest form of sugar, called glucose, which is the key source of energy for the human body. Liver stores glucose and releases it into the bloodstream when it is needed by the cells for energy generation. The hormone called insulin carries glucose to the cells where it is converted into energy. When blood glucose level rises, say after a meal, the pancreas produces more insulin so that more glucose may be carried to the cells while maintaining a constant (normal) concentration of blood glucose. To accomplish this, the glucose-carrying insulin binds itself to insulin receptors on the cell membrane. If all the receptors are fully occupied due to too much glucose in the blood, the excess glucose is carried back (by insulin) to the liver for storage. If, on the other hand, the blood glucose level is too low, say due to fasting, the pancreas produces a hormone called glucagon, which signals the liver to release more glucose into the blood. In this way, the liver regulates the blood-glucose concentration and maintains it at an equilibrium state (homeostasis).

When an insufficient amount of insulin is produced in the pancreas, or when the cell's ability to take in glucose is compromised even with a sufficient amount of insulin, the cells will not be supplied with adequate amount of glucose. When the cells are starved of glucose, due to insufficient insulin production in the pancreas, this condition is called Type 1 diabetes. This usually happens because of defective genes. If an insufficient supply of glucose to the cells is due to the body's inability to use insulin properly, it is called Type 2 diabetes. When glucose builds up in the blood, instead of going into cells, the cells are starved of glucose and cannot generate adequate amounts of energy, which the body needs. In Type 2 diabetes, fat, liver, and muscle cells do not respond correctly to insulin, for example, due to the inability of insulin to bind to the cell membrane receptors. This is called insulin resistance. As a result, blood sugar does not easily get into these cells to be used for energy production. When this happens, the cells are starved of sugar, even though the sugar concentration in the blood is excessive.

Most people with Type 2 diabetes are overweight when they are diagnosed. Increased fat concentration makes it harder for the body to use insulin in the correct way, because excess free fatty acids interfere with insulin-receptor-mediated signalling in loose connective fatty tissues, as well as in liver and skeletal muscles. It is believed that the excess free fatty acids have additional toxic effects on the liver and adipose tissues (loose connective fatty tissues). Studies have shown that excess body weight around the waist, caused mainly by poor diet and low physical activity level, increases the chances of getting Type 2 diabetes. Diets rich in saturated animal fat and refined sugar are believed to be the major contributor to the risk of developing the disease, whereas the plant-based and marine-life-based diets are believed to lower the risk. The former represents an abrupt and significant departure from the human traditional diet appropriate to the present stage of human evolution. Again, these findings lend support to the proposition that the greater a food source's evolutionary distance is from the human species, the healthier it is for humans. Plants and marine lives are farther away from humans evolutionarily than are mammals.

(III) Oxidative-Stress-Related Rationale and Evidence

In biological systems of all animal species, the energy required for life is harnessed by burning the nutrients in the mitochondrial inner membrane of the cell, the process known as cellular respiration or oxidative phosphorylation. During this process, the nutrients are broken down, assisted by numerous enzymes, into simpler molecules that can be oxidized (burned). The process of oxidation involves the transfer of electrons from a substrate to an oxidizing agent. Oxidation reactions can produce what is known as oxygen radicals or free radicals. A free radical is an atom or a group of atoms with an odd (unpaired) number of electrons. Once formed, these highly reactive radicals can start a chain reaction. The chain reaction can be highly damaging to the important cellular components such as DNA or the cell membrane. Cells may function poorly, abnormally, or die if this occurs. It is akin to metals rusting when exposed to oxygen. The free radicals formed during the oxidation process of nutrients inflict corrosive damages to cells. Free radicals are not inherently bad. It is believed that they are involved in inter-cellular and intracellular signalling, and that some oxygen radicals kill invading pathogens. Excessive amounts of free radicals, however, can be extremely damaging to cells.

To prevent free-radical damage, the body has a self-defence system of antioxidants. Antioxidants are molecules that can safely interact with oxygen radicals and terminate the chain reaction. They do this by being oxidized themselves. There are enzymes within the body that scavenge free radicals for this purpose. This self-defence system of the body can be further strengthened through dietary intake of antioxidants such as vitamin E, beta-carotene, and vitamin C. (Beta-carotene is converted to vitamin A in the body.) Usually the body's self-defence system is not sufficient to stop the free-radical chain reactions, particularly when the diet is rich in substance conducive to free-radical formation.

Although as a general rule, oxygen is required in metabolizing the nutrients (aerobic metabolism), this is not always the case. In situations where oxygen is unavailable or scarce, for example, during intensive physical exercise with an insufficient supply of oxygen through the lungs, the metabolism of nutrients without oxygen (anaerobic metabolism) takes over to convert the nutrients to energy. Anaerobic metabolism is a faster (but inefficient) process than aerobic process. The anaerobic process, being inefficient, generates more wastes per calorie of energy produced and alters the pH (acidity) of blood, causing fatigue, and thus is employed only in emergencies where a fast metabolic process is required. After all, this is an ancient metabolic process that our ancestor cells invented 3.5 billion years ago, when oxygen was virtually nonexistent. In the present environment, where oxygen is abundantly available, our body uses a slow but more efficient process of aerobic metabolism.

Although oxidation reactions are crucial for life in aerobic metabolic processes, they can also be highly damaging. Excessive amounts of free radicals can lead to cell injury and death, which can cause many diseases and disorders. Insufficient levels of antioxidants, or the inhibition of antioxidant enzymes, cause oxidative stress. Oxidative stress plays a significant role in many human diseases, including many types of cancer. It is known that oxidative DNA damage is responsible for many types of cancer development (unregulated cell growth). The majority of cancers are believed to be caused by mutations in the DNA, which alter the cell's perception of growth-stimulator signals and push the cell to move to the G1 (growth) phase of the cell cycle. Every cell contains a nucleus made up of nucleic acids, including DNAs and RNAs. When DNA is damaged by the corrosive effect of oxidative stress, the genetic information contained in the DNA is altered. Alteration of the genetic information can cause incorrect signals to be sent to the cell. Wrong signals sent to the cell may also be caused by a damage done to the cell membrane, which controls information flows between the exterior and interior environments of the cell. A typical way in which oxidative stress causes cancer development is through oxidative damage to either DNA or the cell membrane, which alters the signal for cell growth.

Oxidative stress is also believed to contribute to the development of a wide range of other diseases, including Alzheimer's, Parkinson's, diabetes, rheumatoid arthritis, and many motor-neuron diseases, as well as cardiovascular disease. Low-density lipoprotein (LDL) oxidation is believed to trigger the process of atherosclerosis, which can lead to cardiovascular disease. Oxidative stress is also known to negatively affect the body's immune system.

Studies have confirmed that poor diet and an unhealthy lifestyle contribute significantly to oxidative stress. It is known that substances that contribute to oxidative stress include the following: toxic chemical compounds and pollutants, hydrogenated fats, oils heated to high temperatures, too much refined sugar, too much animal protein, preservatives and pesticides in food, drugs (over the counter and prescription), alcohol, cigarette smoke, radiation exposure, and psychological and emotional stress. On the other hand, diets high in fruits and vegetables have been shown to contain high amounts of antioxidants.

Studies have also found that a low-calorie diet extends median and maximum life span in many animals. This effect may involve a reduction in the oxidative stress associated with a low-calorie diet and the associated reduced level of metabolic activities. The evidence also suggests that, in humans, diets high in fruits and vegetables, which are high in antioxidants, promote health and reduce the effects of aging. It is known that excessive amounts of free radicals contribute to premature aging.

A recent study focusing on women has found that diets rich in fruits, vegetables, and berries significantly slow down the process of aging. It is believed that flavonoids (richly contained in fruits, vegetables, and berries) are powerful antioxidants, preventing free-radical damage to cells. Evidence suggests that flavonoids also decrease inflammation, relax blood vessels, and help prevent blood clots that could lead to heart attack or stroke. As well, flavonoids have been shown to activate the brain's natural house-cleaning process, helping remove toxins and other compounds that can interfere with cognitive function. Again, these findings add further support to the proposition that there exists a positive relationship between a food source's evolutionary distance from the human species and its beneficial health effects on humans. Vegetables, fruits, and berries that contain rich amounts of antioxidants are farther distanced evolutionarily from the human species than are the animals whose meat is a major contributor to oxidative stress when consumed by humans.

Further, it is worth reminding ourselves that most of the diseases linked to oxidative stress are those associated with the lifestyle of the modern industrial and information age. The diet, physical activity level, and state of mind associated with this lifestyle are all conducive to oxidative stress. That is, the real culprit behind the pervasiveness of oxidative stress is the abrupt and massive shocks to our living environment caused by the accelerating pace of industrialization and technological change.

(IV) Blood pH-Related Rationale and Evidence

A liquid that has a pH of 7 is considered to be neutral, neither acidic nor alkaline. Pure water has a pH of 7. A liquid with a pH less than 7 is acidic. A liquid with a pH greater than 7 is alkaline. Our blood plasma needs to maintain a pH of 7.35 to 7.45 for the cells to function properly. If the blood pH shifts outside of this range, serious problems can develop in our body, even death. As our cells produce energy on a continual basis, a number of different acids are formed and released into our body fluids. Our body has three major mechanisms at work to tightly regulate and prevent the pH of our blood from being shifted outside of the 7.35 - 7.45 range: (1) buffering systems; (2) exhalation of carbon dioxide; (3) elimination of hydrogen ions through the kidneys. These mechanisms ensure the slightly alkaline level of our blood pH that our body desires. (Readers may consult, for example, http://drbenkim.com for further discussion.)

The pH of blood could fall below 7.35 for a number of reasons, including dietary. This condition is referred to as acidosis. Signs and symptoms that may be seen in acidosis include headaches, confusion, feeling tired, tremors, sleepiness, and dysfunction of the cerebrum of the brain, which may progress to coma if there is no intervention. Since our blood pH should be maintained slightly alkaline, and since our normal diet consists mainly of foods that are acid-forming, it is a good idea to avoid making our diet unnecessarily acid-forming. If your diet consists mainly of foods that are acid-forming, and such a diet is maintained on a sustained basis, chances are that you will overwork the buffering systems to a point where undesirable changes in your health may result. Since your buffering systems have to work all the time in any case, to neutralize the acids that are formed from every day metabolic activities, it is desirable to maintain a diet that doesn't create unnecessary additional work for your buffering systems.

Of particular interest in this context is that, since one of the buffering systems makes extensive use of calcium phosphate salts, which are structural components of bones and teeth, if your body is regularly exposed to large quantities of acid-forming foods and liquids on a sustained basis, your body will have to draw on its calcium-phosphate reserves to supply your phosphate-buffering system, in order to neutralize the acid-forming effects of your diet. Over time, this may lead to structural weakness in your bones and teeth. Drawing on calcium phosphate reserves at a high rate can also increase the amount of calcium that is eliminated through urine, thereby increasing the risk of developing calcium-rich kidney stones.

Most vegetables and fruits have alkaline-forming effects on our body fluids, while animal-based foods and highly processed foods have acid-forming effects. Again, the proposition that there exists a positive relationship between a food source's evolutionary distance from the human species and its beneficial health effects on humans is further supported by these findings. Vegetables and fruits are farther distanced evolutionarily from humans than are animals.

(V) Health Effects of Abrupt and Massive Shocks to the Way Food is Grown, Raised, Processed, and Prepared

Quite apart from the kinds of food humans eat, the way food is grown, raised, processed, prepared, and cooked may have profound effects on human health. Excessive use of pesticides in growing crops, use of certain feeds in raising animals, excessive use of preservatives and other chemicals in food processing, excessive refining of grains and sugar, and intensive cooking (e.g., excessive frying and barbecuing) can all affect adversely the health of the consumers. All of these represent abrupt and massive shocks to the human diet from the evolutionary point of view. Studies show that pesticides, preservatives, and other toxic chemical compounds and pollutants contained in the food, excessive refining of grains and sugar and oils heated in high temperatures all contribute to oxidative stress.

Excessive refining of grains and sugar represent an abrupt and massive departure from the gradual process of human-evolutionary adaptation. When grains are refined, the bran and the germ are removed, along with many valuable nutrients, vitamins, minerals, and dietary fibre they contain. More than that, harmful chemicals may be added in the refining process. A loaf of white bread is sometimes dubbed "a loaf of chemicals." White bread is excessively starchy, virtually devoid of natural fibre, and contains numerous chemicals in the form of bleaches, additives, preservatives, dough conditioners, etc. that are harmful to the human body. Also, vitamins and minerals having been removed, the refined grain products, such as white rice, white flour, white bread, and white pasta will have strong acid-producing effects inside our body, overburdening the body's buffering systems of counteracting acidosis.

They are also nutritionally imbalanced. Altered phosphorus-calcium balance in these products is known to cause calcium leaching from the bones and teeth. It is understood that refined sugar and refined grain products are primarily responsible for tooth decay, as well as being the major cause of brittle bones in the elderly in the industrialized world. In the process of refining sugar, for example, sulfur dioxide is used to bleach the sugar and turn it white, and other chemicals are added, including calcium hydroxide to remove impurities. Raw (brown) sugar, on the other hand, is made by a co-crystallization process that helps it preserve its colour, flavour, and nutrients. In this process, unlike the refining process, the sugar cane is pressed to release its juices, from which the sugar crystals are formed. Unlike the refining process, no nutrients are lost and no chemicals are added during this process.

The starch from excessively refined grains (Amylopectin) is structurally highly branched, leaving more surface area available for digestion, and hence is broken down quickly in the digestive tracts, producing a large increase in blood sugar and subsequently a large, quick rise in insulin. The starch from whole grains (Amylose), on the other hand, is a straight chain, which limits the amount of surface area exposed for digestion, and so is digested more slowly. It is less likely to spike blood sugar and insulin. In fact, this form of starch is not fully digested and absorbed until it makes its way to the large intestine, where it is fermented by intestinal bacteria. This implies that excessively refined grain and sugar products bypass a large part of the natural digestive and absorptive system of the human body and thereby weaken these critically important body organs and their functions, quite apart from the problems the sudden spike in blood sugar and insulin may cause.

Carbonated soft drinks, a major source of fluid intake in the modern affluent society, are another example of extremely undesirable food processing. Most carbonated soft drinks not only contain excessive amounts of refined sugar but are extremely acidic. Most of them have a pH of 3, making them about ten thousand (10^4) times more acidic than pure water! [Note: $10^{7-3} = 10^4$] Although it must be admitted that our body's buffering system is powerful enough to maintain homeostatic blood pH on a constant basis, even with daily consumption of strongly acid-forming foods and drinks, it nevertheless follows that it is desirable to avoid overburdening the buffering systems as much as possible.

In this chapter so far, we have examined the four different areas of human physiology, namely blood cholesterol, insulin resistance, oxidative stress, and blood pH, to see whether abrupt and massive shocks to the diet cause significant damage to human health. In all of the four areas of human physiology examined above, we find that abrupt and massive shocks to our diet seriously damage human health. We have also examined the adverse health effects of abrupt and massive shocks to the way food is grown, raised, processed, prepared, and cooked. Of particular interest to us is that the proposition of positive relationship between a food source's evolutionary (genetic) distance from the human species and its beneficial effects on human health is strongly supported by both our theoretical knowledge and empirical findings. We have found this to be the case in all of the four major areas of human physiology examined. Although we have not explored other areas of human physiology specifically for this purpose, it would not be surprising if we did find further evidence supporting the proposition emerging from research in other areas, considering the fact that the four areas we have examined constitute the key areas of our understanding of human physiology.

B. Abrupt and Massive Shocks to the Level of Physical Activity

The modern industrial and information society has brought about what amounts to an abrupt and massive environmental shock to the human physical-activity level. This has drastically reduced the average level of physical activity for humans with grave health consequences. It has been observed in extensive studies that increasing physical activity can lower blood-cholesterol levels, for instance, and therefore reduce the risk of heart disease and stroke. It stands to reason that increased physical inactivity due to abrupt and massive changes in work environments, caused by the technological change in the modern industrial and information age, contributes to the heightened risk of heart disease and stroke. Studies have also found that low physical-activity levels contribute to the risk of insulin resistance through accumulation of excess free fatty acids in the body, as noted previously. Insulin resistance leads to Type 2 diabetes. Additionally, low physical-activity levels in general cause both physical and mental fitness levels to decrease and the body's immune system to weaken.

While the health benefits of regular and steady physical exercise (appropriate to an individual's age and existing physical-fitness level) cannot be overemphasized, the danger of excessive irregular physical activity must also be recognized. Extensive studies have found that excessive irregular physical exercise contributes to oxidative stress by causing excessive amount of free radicals to be formed, more than the antioxidant defence system can handle, as cellular respiration is ramped up. Regular and steady moderate physical exercise, however, has been shown to reduce oxidative-stress levels by strengthening antioxidant defences. Apparently, free radicals that are formed as a result of initial physical exercise act as a signal for the antioxidant defence system to make necessary adaptations for combating future free radicals and strengthen its defence capabilities. In fact, regular and steady moderate exercises have been found to be associated with decreased free-radical formation, whereas irregular, excessive exercises have been found to be associated with oxidative stress.

C. Abrupt and Massive Shocks to the State of Mind

The modern technology-driven industrial and information society has produced a working environment that makes it difficult for an average worker to be close to nature and maintain a peaceful and cheerful mind. Numerous studies have confirmed, however, that lifestyle stress can lead to various health problems. For example, emotional stress can lead to high blood pressure and an increased risk of heart disease and stroke. When stressed, the body elicits the fight and flight responses by releasing stress hormones such as adrenaline and cortisol into the bloodstream. These stress hormones mobilize fats and cholesterol into the bloodstream to be used by the muscles. When cholesterol content in the blood becomes excessive due to excessive stress, this can lead to high blood pressure and arterial blockage.

It has also been found that chronic release of cortisol, caused by emotional stress, weakens the activity of the immune system. Excessive cortisol also causes breakdown of protein and fat into glucose, thereby elevating the glucose level in the blood and thus increasing the risk of developing Type 2 diabetes. Studies have also confirmed that emotional stress significantly increases free-radical load on the body, as stress induces the release of hormones, such as adrenaline and cortisol. This creates biochemical changes, which increase free-radical stress in the body. Corroborating this, higher protective antioxidant enzyme levels and lower oxidized lipid levels in blood samples of meditation practitioners have been found. Extensive studies have also revealed similar findings for animals.

These findings support the proposition that healthy diet must go hand in hand with adequate levels of physical activity and a stress-free lifestyle (triad equilibrium), if it is to have a maximum salutary effect on healthy living for humans.

VI. Seven Principles For Healthy Living

OUR DISCUSSIONS SO FAR ON THE EVOLUTION OF THE human species, particularly of its diet, physical activity level, and mental and emotional stress level, combined with the theoretical and empirical findings in the four related areas of human physiology, lead us to postulate certain principles for healthy living for humans. I present the following seven principles as a natural outgrowth from our discussions so far:

1. Healthy living starts with working towards a healthy body and mind.

2. A healthy body and mind is achieved through a healthy, balanced diet, an appropriate amount of physical exercise, and maintaining a peaceful and cheerful mind.

3. A healthy, balanced diet is best achieved through the intake of a variety of foods from a variety of

sources, preferably plant and marine-life based, in as natural a state as possible.

4. How much one eats is not as critical for human health as what one eats.

5. The appropriate amount of physical exercise depends on one's age and the existing level of physical fitness.

6. A peaceful and cheerful mind is attained through self-respect, respect for others, respect for nature, a positive attitude toward life, and occasional quiet moments.

7. The ideal body weight is the one associated with one's optimum physical and mental fitness, not a specific number on a scale.

These seven principles for healthy living are discussed in greater detail and depth in the following pages.

The root of all health is in the brain.
The trunk of it is in emotion.
The branches and leaves are the body.
The flower of health blooms
when all parts work together.

~ *Kurdish folk wisdom*

Principle 1. Healthy Living Starts With Working Towards A Healthy Body And Mind.

As the Kurdish folk wisdom cited above suggests, physical health goes hand in hand with mental health. A person without a healthy body cannot have a healthy mind. A person without a healthy mind cannot have a healthy body either. Body and mind support each other to form a unified whole in a state of harmony. One needs the other to be healthy and to stay healthy. Mental health suffers if the body deteriorates and physical health suffers if the mind is not in a harmonious state. A healthy body and healthy mind go together hand in hand, and mutually reinforce each other. Interdependence between the health of body and mind is well accepted by the medical profession. Studies have shown that higher protective anti-oxidant enzyme levels and lower oxidized lipid levels were found in blood samples of meditation practitioners. In a reverse situation, a sick body and a sick mind harm each other in a mutually reinforcing downward spiral. Too often we find that the instances of too much emotional strain result in bodily sicknesses such as cancer.

Scientific research has shown that emotional stress weakens the body's immune system. Emotional stress increases free radical load on the body, as stress induces the release of adrenaline and cortisol hormones, which mobilize the body ready for action, known as the fight and flight responses. This creates biochemical changes, which increase oxidative stress in the body. Oxidative stress can lead to cell membrane and DNA damages, causing a wide range of illnesses including cancer, cardiovascular disease, diabetes, rheumatoid arthritis, Alzheimer's, Parkinson's, and motor-neuron diseases. Emotional stress can also cause bile acid indigestion.

Similarly, a prolonged physical ailment will inevitably negatively impact the state of the mind. In essence, the mind is nothing more than a totality of information about the environment, which we call experience, that the brain perceives through the nerve system, and then processes, stores, and retrieves on an ongoing basis. The totality of information includes what has been accumulated and stored in the DNA throughout the evolutionary time since the beginning of life on earth, as well as the information accumulated and stored during the individual's lifetime. Mind has two components, thinking and feeling. Our brain's ability to think and feel is a natural extension from our brain's ability to gather, process, store, and retrieve this information. (It is our brain, not our heart, that feels, contrary to common perception.) It is then only natural and inevitable that the body and the mind cannot be separated as distinct parts of life. They are integral parts of the whole. In fact, this could be said for other species, not just human.

Life can be quite stressful in the modern, technology-driven world, with its ever-accelerating pace of life. A typical day for a typical working man or woman may look like this. They are woken up in the morning by an alarm clock that has no sympathy, take a quick shower, eat breakfast in a great hurry, fight the morning rush hour traffic (stressful), sit at a desk checking emails (new work generated, deadlines imposed), go to a meeting (more work generated, more deadlines imposed), have lunch (most likely composed of too much unhealthy food), sit at a desk working to meet deadlines (stressful), go home fighting the afternoon rush hour traffic (stressful), have dinner (again most likely containing too much unhealthy food), and sit in front of a TV, munching on unhealthy snacks. This routine is repeated day after day with only minor variations. Only rarely will some amount of physical exercise be thrown in here and there. Some of us who are lucky may find some time for hobbies, entertainment, and social hours, but not nearly sufficient.

Our bodies, a product-in-process of gradual evolutionary adaptation through the ages, are not conditioned for this type of living and working environment, which is vastly different from the one that even our parents and grandparents were conditioned for – never mind the earlier generations. Our living and working environment is changing too fast for the human body and mind to adapt. Too much stress on the mind causes the body to crumble. An unhealthy body causes the mind to lose strength. A downward spiral of deteriorating body and mind may ensue. It takes a great amount of effort and determination to arrest and reverse this downward spiral. Once the downward spiral has been arrested, and made to turn in the opposite direction, a virtuous circle of healthy body and mind can be established. Once established, maintaining the virtuous circle assisted by its momentum would be much easier.

"Sit loosely on the saddle of life."

~ Robert Louis Stevenson

Principle 2. A Healthy Body And Mind Is Achieved Through A Healthy, Balanced Diet, An Appropriate Amount Of Physical Exercise, And Maintaining A Peaceful And Cheerful Mind.

A healthy, balanced diet, an appropriate amount of physical exercise, and a peaceful and cheerful mind are the three essential ingredients, or the triad, for attaining and maintaining mental, emotional, and physical fitness.

They come in a package. All three are necessary. If one is missing, all fall apart. However, with any two of the three well under control, it is a lot easier to accomplish the third. For example, when a healthy, balanced diet and an appropriate amount of physical exercise are achieved and well entrenched, a peaceful and cheerful mind is attainable with relative ease. On the other hand, if for some reason emotional strain persists for an extended period of time, neither a healthy, balanced diet nor the proper amount of physical exercise may be sustainable. When the package of three, or the triad, has been successfully attained and solidified with each component supporting the other two, it is extremely difficult for any external force to break or destabilize it. This is because of a physical phenomenon known as inertia. It is a kind of gravitational pull on each one by the others. However, there may be situations where, although two of the three are well entrenched and the third component is lacking, the package does not unravel quickly. For example, a young person may be able to sustain a reasonable degree of physical fitness with a minimum of physical exercise if strongly supported by a healthy, balanced diet and a peaceful and cheerful mind. For obvious reasons, it is much easier for a younger person to attain and maintain a healthy body and mind than it is for an older person. As one gets older, however, it becomes imperative that all three components support each other. Older persons derive far greater benefits from the triad equilibrium than do younger persons. In fact, it could be said that the benefits of the triad equilibrium increase at an accelerating rate rather than at a constant rate as one gets older.

Living in harmony with nature will make it easier for all of the three components of the triad to support each other in a state of self-sustaining equilibrium. Living in harmony with nature means ensuring that the body and mind are not subjected to sudden, excessive, and prolonged harmful external shocks (in an evolutionary sense), particularly the ones generated by the unnatural, man-made changes to the environment. We have seen in the previous chapter how abrupt and massive environmental shocks to our diet, physical activity level, and state of mind can destroy our health through increases in blood LDL cholesterol, insulin resistance, oxidative stress, and blood acidity. The triad equilibrium will ensure that our lifestyle is minimally affected by such environmental shocks.

> "It is no accident that we see green almost wherever we look ... Without green plants to outnumber us at least ten to one there would be no energy to power us."
>
> ~ Richard Dawkins (*us = non-plant species)

Principle 3. A Healthy, Balanced Diet Is Best Achieved Through The Intake Of A Variety Of Foods From A Variety Of Sources, Preferably Plant And Marine-Life Based, In As Natural A State As Possible.

All living organisms are made up of four classes of large biological molecules: carbohydrates, lipids, proteins, and nucleic acids. The basic building blocks of the cell are sugars that make up carbohydrates, fatty acids that make up lipids, amino acids that make up proteins, and nucleotides that make up nucleic acids. Within cells, these small organic molecules are joined together to form larger molecules. These building blocks of the cell are extracted from the nutrients contained in the foods that we eat. Only some of the foods we eat are broken down into nutrients and burned as fuels. What's not used as fuels are used as starting materials in making DNAs, RNAs, and the proteins and fats that go into the cell membrane.

The cell is the simplest collection of matter that can live. There are two kinds of cells, prokaryotic and eukaryotic. Bacteria and archaea consist of prokaryotic cells. All other living organisms, including all plants and animals (including humans) consist of eukaryotic cells. All cells are descendants of earlier cells. Each cell has its own DNAs (deoxyribonucleic acids) that contain its own genetic information, which is translated by RNAs (ribonucleic acids) for synthesizing proteins, with help from an enzyme called ribosome. Every animal cell has the mitochondrion, the site of cellular respiration, where nutrients are oxidized and converted into energy. Every plant or algae cell has chloroplast, the site of photosynthesis, where the energy from the sunlight is converted into chemical energy in the form of sugar. Mitochondria and chloroplasts are very similar in structure and in form, as well as in metabolic process, which is again similar to the metabolic process of bacteria. Furthermore, every mitochondrion and every chloroplast has its own DNAs, separate from the DNAs of the cell housing it. This has led scientists to believe that both mitochondria and chloroplasts originate from bacteria's metabolic system and that bacteria entered the cells of the plants and animals as parasites in the very early stage of evolution. (Bacteria have their own DNAs.) This is hardly surprising considering the fact that all cells, prokaryotic and eukaryotic, are the descendants of the first ancestor cell. The cells, the most basic components of all living organisms, have apparently kept their original process of metabolizing nutrients basically intact through billions of years of evolutionary time, regardless of whatever species of life they happen to serve as basic components. In fact, a striking feature of metabolism is the similarity of the basic metabolic pathways and components between vastly different species, ranging from unicellular bacterium to huge multicellular organism like the elephant. This is only one of many indications that evolution is a fact of life, rather than just a theory or a hypothesis. Proper understanding of human physiology and human wellness issues would be unthinkable outside the general framework of human evolutionary history.

The foods humans eat today have evolved over billions of years of life's existence. Today's human diet has come to comprise a great variety of foods, ranging from plant material to animal-based foods. This variety is uniquely human. A healthy, balanced diet ensures that our body receives all the nutrients, vitamins, minerals, dietary fibre, and fluid required for maintaining a healthy body and mind in the proper amounts. A healthy, balanced diet is best achieved through the intake of a variety of foods from a variety of sources in as natural a state as possible. One of the reasons why the human species has been able to occupy the present position as a dominant and thriving life form on earth has to do with its diet, which comprises a great variety of food sources. The human diet comprising a great variety of food sources ensures a wide range of dietary choices for humans, lessening the degree of their dependence on a few selected food sources for nutrition. Although a great variety of edible food sources are available to humans, their primary food sources should preferably be plant and marine-life based to the highest extent possible. The reasons for this have been provided in Chapter V, with strongly supporting scientific evidence. Generally speaking, foods we eat should be in as natural a state as possible. Food in a natural state is food left uncooked, unprocessed, or unrefined. Needless to say, food does not have to be in a completely natural state to be eaten. The less-intensely cooked, processed, or refined, however, the higher nutritional and fibre content a food will have – as a general rule, with some exceptions. Also, the less that food is processed, the fewer preservatives and other harmful chemical compounds it is likely to contain. Organically grown or organically raised foods in general are healthier than non-organic foods, as the former contain fewer harmful chemicals. However, even the organic foods, if they are excessively refined, processed, or cooked, may become less healthy than the less intensively refined, processed, or cooked non-organic. How food is prepared matters a great deal.

Food sources should span as wide a range as possible, including grains, cereals, seeds, beans, peas, potatoes, yams, sweet potatoes, plant roots such as carrots, turnips, beets, nuts of all kinds, berries of all kinds, fruits of all kinds, leafy vegetables, legumes, tomatoes, cucumbers, zucchinis, onions, garlic, squashes, pumpkins, melons, broccolis, Brussel sprout, cauliflowers, a variety of sea vegetables, natural honey, brown sugar, vegetable oils, spices, coffee, tea, and so forth. The list is endless. Call this List A. For most people who are not vegetarians, however,

List A is not enough to satisfy their palates. For them the list may be extended to include red meat, poultry, fish, shellfish, calamari, escargots, eggs, dairy products, and so on. Call this list of animal-based foods List B. Finally, we need to drink fluids to supplement what is already supplied through the consumption of fruits, vegetables, and other foods.

Table I. List of Essential and Supplemental Sources of Nutrients

A: Essential Sources of Nutrients	B: Supplemental Sources of Nutrients
Grains, cereals, seeds	Ocean fish
Beans, peas, lentil	Shellfish
Plant roots	Calamari, octopus
Nuts	Fresh water fish
Berries	Eggs
Fruits	Poultry
Vegetable fruits	Wild animal meat
Legumes	Milk & other dairy products
Leafy vegetables	Red meat
Other vegetables	
Sea vegetables	
Natural honey	
Vegetable oils	
Spices	

Note: Readers will find that the above lists are by no means exhaustive.

Both List A and List B items are shown in Table I. Normally List A provides all essential nutrients required for maintaining a healthy human body and mind. For most people, however, it may be necessary to satisfy their palates with an intake of items from List B. Generally speaking, List B items are not as healthy as those on List A. List B items are listed in a descending order of desirability in terms of their benefit to human health. For items on List B, notice the positive relationship between the desirability for human health and the evolutionary distance (or genetic distance) from the human species. Some may wonder whether shellfish such as shrimps, lobsters, and scallops (popularly blamed for high dietary cholesterol) are in fact healthier than other animal meat and dairy products. It is now well known that shellfish contain less dietary cholesterol than dairy products and meat. Furthermore, we know from Chapter V that it is not the high dietary cholesterol but the high saturated fat content in a food that is responsible for high LDL cholesterol in the blood. It is known that shellfish are significantly lower in saturated fats and significantly higher in polyunsaturated fats than other animal meat and dairy products. Shellfish also contain significant amounts of other non-cholesterol sterols that can decrease the absorption of cholesterol in the body. Recent studies have shown that Chinese men who consumed fish or shellfish weekly had significantly reduced odds of having a heart attack. We have also seen in Chapter V that eggs, high in dietary cholesterol, do not contribute to the raising of blood LDL cholesterol for the same reason. Eggs, however, do not contain some of the beneficial nutrients that shellfish do.

As a general rule, the farther away the nutritional source is from the human species in terms of evolutionary distance, the greater is its desirability in terms of its benefit to human health and vice versa. Persuasive scientific evidence for this proposition, both theoretical and empirical, has been provided in Chapter V. This of course makes perfect sense when viewed in light of the survival of the species in the context of the theory of evolution. Viewed in this light it may be concluded that human meat is the most harmful to human health and the meat of the primates is the next most harmful. If this weren't the case, it would have been difficult for biology to repudiate cannibalism! The evolutionary logic implies that it is not in the species' best interest to eat its own meat. Furthermore, the logic also implies that eating the meat of close evolutionary cousins is not as healthy as eating the meat of distant evolutionary relations. It naturally implies that List A items are healthier foods for humans than List B items, since the former are evolutionarily farther from the human species than the latter. After all, all nutrients originate from the sugar manufactured by green plants through the mechanism of photosynthesis. Animals cannot manufacture nutrients. Animals have acquired, over time, in the course of evolution, the ability to digest plants and subsequently other animals.

We have seen in previous chapters that scientific research findings are virtually unanimous in condemning saturated fat, contained in animal meat, dairy products, lard, and shortening as contributing to elevated levels of LDL cholesterol in blood, which can damage artery walls, while praising healthy unsaturated fat, contained in fish such as salmon, mackerel, tuna, or fat-containing vegetables, such as avocados, nuts and seeds, and vegetable oils. Unsaturated fats contained in the latter have been found to counteract the LDLs by increasing HDLs that carry excess LDLs back to the liver, thereby preventing damage to the artery walls. Studies have also confirmed that diets high in fruits and vegetables are high in antioxidants, which inhibit oxidation reactions that produce cell-damaging free radicals, while diets high in animal protein, refined sugar, hydrogenated fats, and processed foods contribute to oxidative stress. Oxidative stress can cause damages to cell membrane and DNA, which can lead to a variety of diseases, including cancer. Scientific evidence is equally strong that vegetables and fruits have alkaline-forming effects on our body fluids, whereas animal-based foods, highly processed foods, and carbonated soft drinks have acid-forming effects. Since our body's buffering system has to work constantly to neutralize the acids that are formed from everyday metabolic activities to maintain appropriate blood pH, it is in our best interest not to add additional acids to our bloodstream but to follow a diet that does not create unnecessary work for the body's buffering system. The list of findings that support the proposition of a positive relationship between a food source's evolutionary distance from the human species and its benefits to human health seems endless.

Humans may be omnivores but their natural diet at the present stage of their evolution may primarily be plant and marine-life based. The shape and alignment of human teeth also support this proposition (Nathaniel Dominy). Perhaps even stronger supporting evidence for this proposition is the fact that humans cannot survive very long by eating List B items alone, although they are perfectly capable of surviving and prospering on a diet consisting primarily of List A items, supplemented by upper echelon List B items. This line of reasoning suggests that the ideal diet for humans should consist primarily of List A items, supplemented by the items in the upper echelon of List B. However, if one needs to include the lower echelon List B items in a diet, for whatever reason, he or she is advised to avoid the items at the very bottom of the list as much as possible.

Should you wish to confine your diet to List A items only, it is important that as many varied items as possible are included, ideally covering the entire range of foods within the list over some period of time. The variety ensures that all necessary nutrients are obtained, including essential vitamins and minerals in sufficient quantities. Within List A, you can eat or drink as much or as often as you feel like as long as your stomach feels comfortable, provided that you observe the following guidelines:

1. Stay away from fast foods if at all possible.

2. Stay away from deep-fried foods.

3. Try to avoid highly processed foods as much as possible.

4. For desserts, eat fresh or dried fruit. Avoid pies, cakes, or other baked goods as much as possible.

5. Stay away from sweets such as candies, chocolate bars, brownies, tarts, etc. as much as possible.

6. Try to avoid salty foods.

7. Avoid carbonated soft drinks and energy drinks if at all possible.

8. Black coffee is fine, but green tea is preferable.

9. Avoid excessive consumption of alcoholic beverages.

10. Drink plain water or filtered water. (In most places, tap water is safe and preferable to bottled water.)

11. Use brown sugar or natural honey instead of refined sugar as a sweetener.

12. Try to avoid eating butter or margarine if at all possible.

13. Do not smoke. (This is not necessarily diet-related advice.)

These guidelines are designed to assist you in minimizing the intake of refined sugar and animal fat (a List B item that creeps in), which are the two worst enemies of good health as we have seen in the previous chapter. The desserts and sweets mentioned above invariably contain too much animal fat in the form of butter and dairy milk, in addition to excessive amounts of refined sugar.

Avoid highly processed and highly refined foods as much as possible. The undesirable health effects of highly refined and processed foods have been thoroughly discussed in the previous chapter. The need to avoid excessive consumption of these types of foods cannot be overemphasized. Highly refined and highly processed foods tend to have excessive amounts of preservatives and other harmful chemicals that overburden our body's inherent capacity to remove toxic compounds. It is critical for maintaining a healthy body that toxic wastes are removed as quickly as possible as soon as they are generated during the normal metabolic processes. Any additional harmful chemicals introduced externally, in the form of preservatives and other chemicals, impose an additional burden on the body's ability to cleanse itself. Harmful substances should be quickly removed, so as not to allow them to inflict serious damages to internal organs and the body itself. All species, including humans, have over time developed, through the process of evolutionary adaptation, certain abilities to cope with adverse external shocks to the system, such as gradual environmental changes or impurities contained in the foods they eat. This self-defence mechanism, or self-purifying mechanism, however, has its limitations. Abrupt and excessive shocks to the system can cause a breakdown of these coping mechanisms and can cause a malfunction of the system in the form of various types of disease. This provides the rationale for preferring natural over refined and processed foods as much as possible. Although consumption of some amounts of processed and refined foods is unavoidable, we should try to limit their consumption to the extent possible. For similar reasons we should keep the air we breathe and the water we drink free of contamination by harmful chemicals.

One of the symptoms of unhealthy diet is obesity. At airports or on city streets around the world, we are struck by what we see. We find that native Asians and native Africans tend to be slimmer than North Americans and Europeans. It doesn't take complex reasoning to recognize that it is mainly their diet that is responsible for the differences in physical shape. Even in Asia and Africa, in those pockets where a Western diet has penetrated, we find obesity becoming an increasing concern. The Western diet is rich in animal fat, dairy products, refined grains, and refined sugar (either lower echelon List B items or refined List A items), whereas the traditional Asian and African diets are primarily plant based, i.e., less animal based. Needless to say, slimness does not equate to physical fitness. Sometimes slimness may suggest malnutrition. That is the reason why a vegetarian diet needs to be carefully chosen to make sure that it is nutritionally balanced. It is not uncommon to see disastrous health consequences of overzealous extreme dieting being reported. In fact, the ideal diet does not have to be completely vegetarian as long as those List B items that are included are restricted primarily to the upper echelon of the list as we have seen in the previous chapter.

> *"You are what you eat."*
>
> ~ Victor Lindlahr

Principle 4: How Much One Eats Is Not As Critical For Human Health As What One Eats.

Healthy weight is a critical indicator of human health. Many health problems are caused by or associated with overweight. Conventional wisdom tells us to burn up more calories than are taken in, in order to lose weight. This is dangerously misleading advice, although the statement itself is mathematically correct. This statement focuses attention on calorie counting rather than on what type of food one should be eating. How much one eats is not as critical for human health as what one eats. As long as your diet is limited to List A items, supplemented perhaps by the items in the upper echelon of List B, it doesn't matter how much you eat, provided that variety is maintained for nutritional balance. In fact, you cannot possibly over-eat List A items. Your body automatically regulates the amount of intake through feelings of hunger. If you are hungry, you eat; if you are not, you don't eat; although a regular eating pattern, whether three meals a day or two meals a day, is desirable. Usually the desired amount of food intake will depend on the amount of physical activity one undertakes. As long as your diet is limited to List A items and possibly to the upper echelon of List B items, there is no need to "diet". You only need to pay attention to the nutritional balance of what you eat, not the amount. Your body – your physically and emotionally healthy body – will tell you how much to eat. A physically active person with strong muscles will want to eat more. A person less physically active, with less muscle mass (although perfectly healthy) will want to eat less.

The primary objective should be to attain and maintain a healthy weight, not to lose weight. Your healthy weight may be greater or less than your current weight depending on whether your current weight is mostly due to body fat or muscle mass. A weight gain resulting from replacing body fat with muscle mass would be a perfectly legitimate and healthy objective.

Attention must be paid not only to what and how much to eat but also to how food is prepared. For example, deep-fried fish may not be healthier than roast chicken even though fish in general is regarded as healthier than chicken. For the same reason, deep-fried chicken (such as chicken wings) may not be healthier than roast beef. Similarly, roast potatoes without butter are healthier than potatoes mashed with butter. The list goes on and on. How food is prepared matters a great deal.

Principle 5: The Appropriate Amount Of Physical Exercise Depends On One's Age And The Existing Level Of Physical Fitness.

The modern-technology-driven lifestyle is an abrupt and extreme aberration from the natural course of gradual human evolutionary adaptation process. This lifestyle does not allow most people sufficient time for an adequate level of physical activity. Lack of physical activity can cause a physical fitness level to deteriorate. "Use it or lose it" is a dictum that eloquently speaks to the importance of the physical exercise required for physical fitness. What is then the appropriate amount of physical exercise? While the importance of an appropriate level of exercise cannot be overemphasized, the harmful effects of over-exercise, particularly sudden and irregular, must also be recognized. There seems to be a popular notion that physical exercise is inherently good and that the more exercise, the better. Nothing could be farther from the truth. While it is true that a sufficient level of physical exercise is critically important for healthy body and mind, it is equally important that a care be taken to avoid the exercise that is too strenuous relative to what your body can tolerate. Too much exercise may be more harmful to the body than no exercise at all in certain circumstances.

During exercise, oxygen consumption drastically increases. This leads to a large increase in the production of oxidants known as free radicals. This triggers activation of the self- defence system of antioxidants to prevent oxidative damage to the cells. A sudden excessive exercise, however, can lead to the presence of excessive oxidants in blood that may be too much for the self-defence system to cope with, and can cause oxidative stress that contributes to muscular fatigue and premature aging of the body. Prolonged oxidative stress can damage cell membrane and DNA with potentially serious consequences, as described in the previous chapter. Studies have found, however, that gradually increasing regular physical exercise actually reduces free-radical load by strengthening the anti-oxidative defence mechanism, whereas sudden and excessive physical exercise increases it. Sudden and excessive physical exercise relative to what your body is accustomed to can tax your body's defence system of antioxidants. As a general rule, the amount and vigour of exercise should decrease as one's age increases, other things being equal. In any case, it should be within the limit set by one's fitness level and diet. The level and amount of physical activities can be increased gradually as the state of physical fitness and the quality of diet improve.

The role of oxygen is a paradox in life. The life of the modern multicellular organism is not possible without oxygen. Oxygen is needed to generate energy to power the activities of life, both physical and mental. Oxygen interacts with the molecules of nutrients to generate the energy needed for life, but free radicals are produced during this process as inevitable byproducts. Free radicals themselves are not necessarily harmful unless present in excessive quantities. Oxygen is indispensable for life, but at the same time can be a chief enemy of life, if allowed to run wild in free-radical chain reactions, damaging vital cell components and thereby causing diseases and premature aging. It is critically important to avoid improper diets and improper exercise habits that could contribute to damaging free-radical chain reactions. Diets high in fruits and vegetables, which are high in antioxidants, can reduce the effects of aging and help prevent the diseases, such as cancer, caused by oxidative stress.

For an apt illustration of an appropriate level of physical exercise, think of the human body as a machine, which it really is. Although there are fundamental differences between an organic life form and an inorganic machine, there still exist many similarities between the two, such as wear and tear and inherent mortality. Compare the human body to an automobile, for example. Both require fuel to function. In both cases, what type of fuel is put in matters a great deal. Highly processed foods and fast foods fed to the human body are like contaminated fuel for an automobile. Both require regular maintenance. In the case of an automobile, all parts must be kept clean and well lubricated, and worn out parts must be replaced to extend its life expectancy, but it must eventually be scrapped. In the case of the human body, the right amount of nutritional intake through a healthy and well-balanced diet, with an appropriate level of physical exercise and mental harmony, maintains the body in a healthy condition, but life comes to an end eventually. In the case of an automobile, driving it constantly and running up the mileage shortens its remaining life expectancy. However, driving it too infrequently or too little also shortens its life span. Similarly in the case of the human body, over-exercise beyond the level that can be endured by a healthy body shortens its remaining life expectancy. Professional athletes who engage in aggressive and strenuous sports are known to have shorter longevity and are prone to have more health problems in later life than the general population. However, an insufficient exercise of the human body also tends to shorten a life span. In both cases, an appropriate level of exercise (driving) with proper maintenance is the key to a healthy and long life. In the case of the human body, due to its organic nature, proper maintenance of the vital organs responsible for food intake, digestion, absorption, circulation, and waste removal is critically important, because poor maintenance impinges on both physical and mental health. In organic life forms, physical health and mental health go together hand in hand. The right amount of physical exercise will help the body to function as a well-calibrated organic life form, capable of constantly replacing dying cells with newly created healthy cells (within limits).

Quite apart from the wear-and-tear effect (oxidative stress effect) of the excessive physical exercise, there may also exist what may be termed the 'biological-clock effect'. Just as it is true that, no matter how well an automobile is maintained, it cannot outlast its maximum life expectancy measured in mileage, it is also the case that, no matter how well a human body and mind is maintained through appropriate diet, physical exercise, and disciplining of the mind, an individual cannot outlive the maximum human life expectancy set by what may be called an evolutionarily or genetically determined biological clock. It is quite possible that excessive physical exercise causes the biological clock to tick faster than otherwise, in a manner similar to running up the mileage of an automobile. It may be that insufficient exercise causes the body parts to rust and shortens the life span, and at the same time excessive exercise runs up the mileage or hastens ticking of the biological clock and shortens the remaining life span whether for a machine or for a person.

> "*Honest concern for others is the key factor in improving our day-to-day lives. When you are warm-hearted, there is no room for anger, jealousy, or insecurity. A calm mind and self-confidence are the basis for happy and peaceful relations with each other.*"
>
> ~ Dalai Lama

Principle 6: A Peaceful And Cheerful Mind Is Attained Through Self-Respect, Respect For Others, Respect For Nature, A Positive Attitude Toward Life, And Occasional Quiet Moments.

In the modern technology-driven industrial and information society, where machines and technological gadgets govern the pace of our lives (a sudden and massive environmental shock from an evolutionary point of view), it is becoming increasingly difficult for humans to maintain (on a daily basis) a peaceful and cheerful mind. This makes it ever more important that we make an extra effort to attain and maintain a peaceful and cheerful mind. The minimum prerequisites for a peaceful and cheerful mind are self-respect, respect for others, and respect for nature. A positive attitude toward life and occasional quiet moments are helpful and desirable. Meditation is not a prerequisite but helps to maintain a peaceful mind. There are many techniques for those who are serious about meditation. But, for most people, deep breathing for 5 – 10 minutes at a time, a few times a day, and occasionally looking up at the sky to relieve the tensions that build up during the course of a day should suffice. One helpful way of maintaining a peaceful mind is what Thich Nhat Hanh (*Savor: Mindful Eating, Mindful Life,* Thich Nhat Hanh and Dr. Lilian Cheung, 2010) calls "mindful living." Mindful living is taking time to appreciate or savour each moment of life: what you see, hear, smell, taste, touch, feel, and think. Mindful living is living each moment fully.

Studies have confirmed that emotional stress drastically increases the presence of free radicals in blood, suggesting that uncontrolled emotional stress can lead to oxidative stress. Studies have also confirmed that higher protective antioxidant enzyme levels and lower oxidized lipid levels were found in blood samples of meditation practitioners. Similar findings for animals have been reported extensively. The health benefits of maintaining a stress-free state of mind have been empirically confirmed by extensive research findings.

Practical tips for keeping a peaceful and cheerful mind suggest themselves. Try not to be bothered by inconsiderate drivers on the road or unfriendly remarks by your co-workers or customers. Be nice to people and smile whenever you can. Try to have fun at work. Enjoy your life. Be thankful for what you have. Excessive greed and envy will ruin your health and rob you of happiness. You will be tested at times. Be strong and keep a positive attitude toward life. There are no obstacles that you cannot overcome with positive and winning attitudes, if you do not let greed and envy blind your vision. Failures are inevitable at times. If you do fail, consider it a valuable lesson.

Most importantly, keep peace with yourself. Be compassionate and generous to others as well as to yourself. Compassion and generosity grow out of self-respect and respect for fellow human beings. Remember that self-respect, respect for others, and respect for nature are the minimum requirements for attaining a peaceful and cheerful mind. Those with deep religious faith – truly inclusive and accepting rather than dogmatic or self-righteous – may have the advantage of having already possessed many of the skills, and the mindset, required for this.

Jeremy Bentham, eighteenth-century, English, utilitarian-philosopher, viewed human beings as pleasure-pain calculating machines, constantly attempting to maximize net pleasure (pleasure minus pain). Pleasure comes from satisfying wants. Pain comes from failing to satisfy wants. The greater the wants, the greater are the chances for failing to satisfy them. Excessive wants are greed. Greed increases chances of pain. A greedy person may never be able to satisfy his/her excessive wants and may, as a consequence, live a painful and miserable life. A person with modest wants, on the other hand, has better chances of having them satisfied and living a satisfied life.

Feeling of loving and being loved is the state of ultimate satisfaction or happiness. To love is to put the needs of your loved one ahead of your own. When the needs of your loved one are met, you are happy. That is love. Love may be the most mysterious and most misunderstood (or "un-understood") of human feelings. Love heals even sickness. A feeling of love improves one's health. Reciprocal love is Utopian. Love even un-reciprocated is better than no love and certainly trumps hatred. One who loves always wins. One who hates always loses. Love does not calculate. In fact, if there is any calculation, love calculates inversely. Love makes your body and mind healthy. It does this in a mysterious way. Failed love can be painful but true love heals it.

Principle 7: The Ideal Body Weight Is The One Associated With One's Optimum Physical And Mental Fitness, Not A Specific Number On A Scale.

When you feel physically fit and emotionally at peace with yourself, your face will radiate beauty and charm. You have attained the ideal body weight. Normally, in such a state, you will look slim. But this may not necessarily be the case, depending on your hereditary or other biological baselines. Regardless, you will feel great about yourself and others around you. You will be happy. And this is what really matters.

Weight gain is not necessarily harmful to the body in all situations. Body weight gained from greater muscle mass rather than additional fat is perfectly healthy and desirable. A muscular person's ideal weight is greater than that of a less muscular person, other things being the same. Simply losing weight should not be a goal in itself. In many situations, a weight gain resulting from replacing body fat with muscle mass would be a perfectly legitimate and healthy objective. Your ideal body weight is whatever happens to be associated with your healthy body and mind. The ideal body weight helps you experience spiritual uplifting and emotional happiness.

VII. Putting The Seven Principles Into Practice

"Ideas without action are worthless."

~ Helen Keller

THE TRIAD OF A HEALTHY, BALANCED DIET, AN APPROpriate amount of physical exercise and a peaceful and cheerful mind is derived from the seven principles for healthy living described above, which are in turn grounded in the notion that a healthy body and mind are best achieved by living in harmony with nature, that is, by respecting the natural process of human evolutionary adaptation. The triad is illustrated in the following diagram.

Figure 1. <u>Triad of a healthy balanced diet, an appropriate amount of physical exercise and a peaceful and cheerful mind</u>

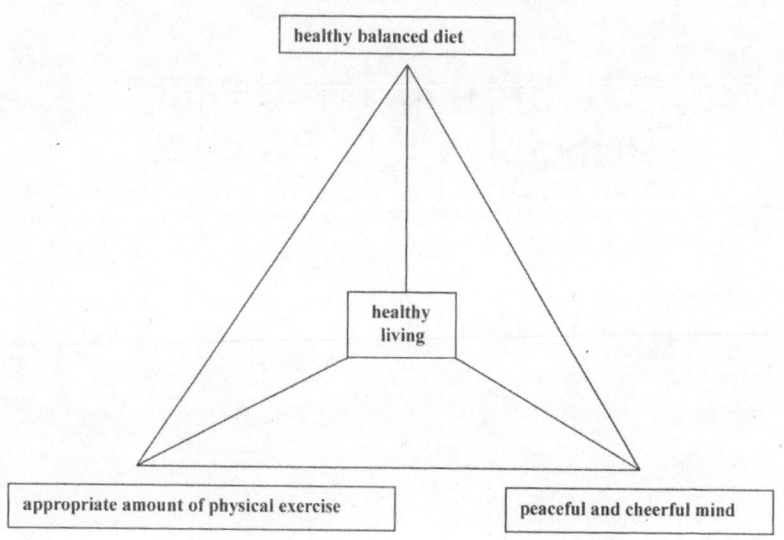

In attaining and maintaining a healthy lifestyle, each of the triad's three components is very important, but since eating is the first requirement for survival, we will start with a discussion about a properly balanced and healthy diet.

A. How To Achieve And Maintain A Properly Balanced, Healthy Diet

We have stated earlier that a healthy, balanced diet is best achieved through the intake of a variety of foods from a variety of sources, preferably plant and marine-life based, in as natural a state as possible. To restate this in specific terms, the requirements for a properly balanced, healthy diet are:

> 1) all the nutrients, vitamins, and minerals required for a healthy human body in appropriate quantities;
>
> 2) the more varied the source of nutrients, the better;
>
> 3) the farther away from the human species the nutrient source is distanced, evolutionarily, the better (e.g., for protein and fat, beans and nuts are better than fish, which is better than poultry, which is better than red meat, and so forth);
>
> 4) the more naturally gown or raised, the better;
>
> 5) the less processed, the better;
>
> 6) the less refined, the better;
>
> 7) the less intensely cooked, the better;
>
> 8) sufficient amount of dietary fibre; and
>
> 9) an adequate amount of fluid.

How much one eats is not as critical for human health as what one eats. As long as you maintain a properly balanced, healthy diet, an appropriate level of physical exercise, and a peaceful and cheerful mind, you can eat as much as your body desires. You cannot possibly over-eat as long as all three components of the triad support each other in an equilibrium state. A common mistake people make in dieting is counting just calories without paying attention to the sources of those calories. What one eats matters more than how much one eats. A rule of thumb is that the ideal amount of food intake in good variety is the one associated with bowel movement once or twice a day with good quality stools. A good quality stool is indicated by an easy and smooth bowel movement, with little or no residue to be wiped off, and with little or no odour. A bowel movement once a day is normal, but with a diet exceptionally rich in fibre, twice in a day is not unusual. In any case, the quality of a stool is a good indicator of whether or not food intake was of the appropriate quantity and quality. Usually, less frequent bowel movements, given the quantity of food intake, indicate less fibre content in a diet and vise versa. Ideally, bowel movements should occur early in the morning, just before or after breakfast.

You will most likely have to go through the following seven steps to achieve and maintain a properly balanced, healthy diet:

Step 1. Assess your present diet.

Step 2. Identify the deficiencies in your present diet.

Step 3. Rectify the deficiencies in stages by setting up intermediate targets.

Step 4. Acquire the taste associated with the new, modified healthier diet.

Step 5. Make the modified healthier diet a habit.

Step 6. Advance to the next stage of an even healthier diet.

Step 7. Repeat steps 3 through 6 until you have reached your final goal.

When you have reached a final goal with which you are happy, you can look back. You will realize that you could never go back to the old diet even if you tried to do so. You have achieved your goal!

Step 1. Assess Your Present Diet.

The first step in achieving a properly balanced, healthy diet is to find out how far your present diet falls short of the desired healthy diet. One way to do this is to write down everything you eat and drink during the course of each day for about two weeks. A table such as the following may be useful for this purpose. Using a table such as this, list each item of food and drink, the quantity consumed, and a brief description of how it was prepared, for each day by time of day, e.g., breakfast, lunch, dinner, snack, etc.

Table II. Assessment of the Present Diet		
For Week of January 5, 2015		
what	how much	brief description
Monday, January 5		
Breakfast:		
Lunch:		
Dinner:		
[Snack]:		

Tuesday, January 6
Breakfast:
Lunch:

(and so on)

Repeat this for each day of the week for at least two weeks, until you get a good sense of what your present diet is like and how far it falls short of your intermediate target diet. The intermediate target diet is any diet that is healthier than your present one, and that you have set for yourself as an intermediate target. Use the positive relationship between a food source's evolutionary distance from the human species, and its desirability for human health, as a guide for setting an intermediate target. Refer to Table I, introduced in the previous chapter, and its accompanying discussion to refresh your memory.

Step 2. Identify the Deficiencies in Your Present Diet.

If you find that your diet contains too much red meat, animal fat, butter and other dairy products, refined sugar, processed food, cakes, pies, fruit juices, soft drinks and energy drinks, try to reduce (to the extent possible) the quantities consumed and gradually work towards the eventual elimination of them from your diet. It is generally known that diet soft drinks are just as bad as regular soft drinks. Carbonated soft drinks are known to be extremely acidic, and in fact 10 thousand times more acidic than pure water! High levels of acidity of blood plasma (acidosis) can cause a variety of health problems as mentioned before. For example, acidosis can lead to osteoporosis and soft teeth, as the body's buffering system tries to restore the blood pH to its normal level by drawing calcium from the bones and teeth. Fruit juices generally contain too much refined sugar. Eat fruits instead. Eat fresh fruits as well as dried fruits. Energy drinks are known to contain brominated vegetable oil and excessive amounts of sugar and caffeine. Bromine can accumulate inside the body and its excessive accumulation can cause skin and nerve damage.

Try to eat vegetables of all shapes and colours. Try to eat whole grain products instead of refined varieties. Try to minimize the consumption of dairy products, with the possible exception of low-fat yogurt and cottage cheese, which contain less fat than other dairy products. Chocolate is beneficial to human health, but the sugar contained in chocolate bars to neutralize the bitter taste is not. Use Table I, and its accompanying discussion, as a guide in determining the deficiencies in your present diet.

The following lists show examples of primary nutrient sources in order of their desirability for human health, suggested by the positive relationship between a food source's evolutionary distance from the human species and its desirability for human health and other requirements for a healthy, balanced diet (stated earlier in this chapter).

Protein

Most desirable:
- nuts, beans, peas, lentil, seeds, whole grains, etc.
- ocean fish
- shellfish, calamari, octopus
- fresh water fish
- escargots
- eggs
- poultry meat
- wild animal meat
- low-fat yogurt, cottage cheese
- low-fat milk

- pork, ham
- beef, lamb
- butter, cheese, hard margarine

Least desirable:
- bacon, sausages, etc.

Carbohydrate

Most desirable:
- whole grains (e.g., wheat, rice, barley, oat, millet, corn)
- roots (e.g., potatoes, yams, sweet potatoes), fruits
- honey, brown sugar
- refined flour (white bread, white pasta), white rice
- crackers, biscuits, etc.

Least desirable:
- deep fried foods (e.g., donuts), baked goods (e.g., muffins, cakes, pies), refined sugar

Fat

Most desirable:
- vegetable oils, nuts, seeds
- fish oil
- eggs
- poultry fat

Least desirable:

– animal fat, dairy milk, other dairy products

Needless to say, the above lists are by no means exhaustive but merely suggestive, and the order of desirability is not exact but only approximate.

Vitamins and minerals:

Most of the desirable sources of protein, carbohydrates, and fat are also rich in the vitamins and minerals needed for human health. In addition, vegetables of all kinds provide essential vitamins and minerals. Leafy vegetables of varied colours and vegetable fruits, such as tomato, squash, cucumber, zucchini, and melon, are good sources of nutrients as well as vitamins and minerals. So also are vegetable roots, such as carrot, beet, turnip, onion, and garlic to name a few. Try to consume a variety of leafy vegetables, vegetable fruits, vegetable roots, and sea vegetables. Sea vegetables are exceptionally rich in iodine and other minerals, and are in general healthier than land vegetables. This obviously reflects the fact that the earliest forms of life originated in the sea. The greater the variety, the better. Fruits of all kinds, fresh or dried, are also a good source of nutrients, vitamins, and minerals. As emphasized earlier, fruits and vegetables are high in antioxidants, as well as alkaline-forming.

Dietary Fibre:

The human body not only needs nutrients, vitamins, and minerals but also needs dietary fibre. Dietary fibre is derived from plant sources, such as fruits, vegetables, and whole grains, and contributes to a healthy diet and lifestyle. Although most fibres are carbohydrates, they cannot be digested by the human body so do not contribute calories to one's diet.

There are two primary types of fibre: soluble fibre and insoluble fibre. Insoluble fibres are like sponges. They absorb and hold water. This enlarges stool and improves bowel movements, thereby helping cleanse the interior walls of the bowels as the contents pass through the colon. Scientific research has shown that this cleansing action may help prevent colorectal cancers and diverticulitis (bacterial infection of the diverticula, tiny pockets in the small intestine). Soluble fibre, such as in fruit pectins and guar gum, have been found to be helpful in preventing atherosclerosis by reducing high cholesterol and triglycerides, thereby decreasing one's risk of heart disease and stroke. Also, foods containing a lot of fibre, such as fruits, vegetables, and whole grain products, slow down digestion of glucose, so they do not cause the sudden insulin spike (and subsequent crash) that refined grain and sugar products cause. That also means the body has more time to use up glucose as fuel before storing it as fat. The slow process of digestion and absorption also means that the entire range of digestive and absorptive organs and functions are fully utilized and as a result strengthened.

Fluid:

Water makes up about 65 percent of the human body, and is vital to the health and functioning of all of our body systems. Lack of water in the body leads to dehydration and can lead to the buildup of toxins. Water plays a critical role in maintaining one's body temperature through perspiration. Water also plays an important role in the digestive process. Saliva, partially composed of water, is the first thing that begins to break down food. Water is needed to break down minerals and soluble fibre in the digestive tracts. Water helps absorb the nutrients and vitamins from foods and release harmful toxins and waste through urine, sweat, and feces.

Hydrated bodies are better at fighting off illness and disease as water is present in the lymph nodes of the immune system. Water keeps skin healthy and prevents the skin disease associated with dehydration. Water keeps our tissue moist and helps protect areas that have thin membranes, such as the mouth, eyes, and nose. Water also lubricates our joints and protects them by adding cushioning around them. Water helps carry oxygen and disperse it throughout the body, bringing nutrients to all parts. It also removes carbon dioxide as it travels through the body.

While adequate hydration is absolutely essential to a properly functioning body, intake of too much water, especially over a short period of time, can be dangerous. If more water enters the body than the kidneys can process, the mineral content of the blood decreases and the overall sodium levels of blood drop. The decrease in sodium and electrolyte levels in the blood causes water to escape the blood and enter the cells to restore electrolyte equilibrium, causing the cells to swell. When this occurs in the brain and when the brain cell swelling is severe enough, it can lead to brain damage, since the brain is housed within the skull with little room to expand – although it would take a huge amount of water intake over a very short period of time for this to occur. In addition, excessive amount of water intake over a very short period of time will add to the body's overall blood volume and put unnecessary strain on the heart and circulatory system.

What is an adequate level of water intake? The U.S. Institute of Medicine recommends 13 cups a day for men and 9 cups a day for women. The exact amount of water that one should consume each day, however, depends on factors such as body weight, level of activity, diet, and age. A rule of thumb is that, given a balanced, healthy diet, one should drink when one feels thirsty. In taking fluid, try to avoid taking it from soft drinks, diet soft drinks, energy drinks, or fruit juices, if at all possible. Carbonated soft drinks, energy drinks and most fruit juices contain too much refined sugar. Energy drinks may also contain bromine, which can accumulate in our bodies over time with harmful consequences. Additionally, most carbonated soft drinks are severely acid-forming, more so than most acid-forming solid foods. Tap water is safer and environmentally friendlier than bottled water. Fluid in the form of plain water or green tea is recommended. Coffee is acceptable, although less desirable in general than green tea or plain water.

Step 3. Rectify the Deficiencies in Stages by Setting up Intermediate Targets.

Eating and drinking habits cannot be changed overnight. It takes time to relinquish the tastes you are accustomed to and to acquire new tastes. Changing a diet requires time and determination, but it can be done and many people have done it successfully. It helps to set intermediate targets and time frames for achieving goals gradually, step by step. Do not expect quick results. Thich Nhat Hanh suggests that, for each intermediate stage, a concrete mission statement be written out, which should be posted in a prominent spot (such as a fridge door) and be looked at periodically as a reminder of the goal to be achieved at that stage. A mission statement may look something like this: "Reduce the amounts taken of butter, refined sugar, animal fat, and soft drinks by 50 percent by January 31." Use whatever system works best for you.

Changing a well-entrenched diet requires determination, a new vision, and most of all, self respect. Self respect comes from the realization that you are a very special person. You are very special, because there is no being exactly like you in the entire universe. Sometimes you may not like the way you look, but then who do you want to look like? Is there someone, some specific person, that you wish you looked like? Not really. If you were given a hypothetical choice between being totally transformed into some specific person and staying as you are at present, you would no doubt want to stay as you are. Most people would. In fact, it is hard to imagine anybody who wouldn't. Being totally transformed into someone else would be tantamount to having yourself killed. Deep down in your mind, you love yourself more than anybody else. That's a biological fact! You are the person you love most despite an appearance that you may not like. That should give you a strong incentive to change your diet, if changing the diet can make you healthier and look more appealing by your own standard.

To be sure, this is easier said than done. For most people, accustomed to a modern way of life, there are numerous hurdles to overcome in achieving and maintaining a healthy, balanced diet. Most people, caught in the fast and hectic pace of life, find it hard to find the time to cook healthy meals every day and to resist the temptation to resort to fast foods and processed foods when a variety of them are easily available and accessible. Even when dining out, healthy meals are not always available. There are also explicit and implicit social pressures to conform to a normal (socially acceptable) lifestyle that are hard to resist. Faced with such enormous hurdles, it is easy for most people to throw in the towel even before leaving the starting gate, or to give up too soon after leaving the gate. In situations like these, however, it is important to set practical intermediate targets that are modest and not too ambitious. Try to make progress in small but steady steps, such as cutting down on butter, sweets, soft drinks, etc., as a first step. Progress builds on progress. Any amount of progress is better than none and certainly better than regress.

Another important thing to keep in mind is that the more physically fit you are, the more efficient will be the digestive, absorptive, circulatory, and waste removal functions of your body, and hence the faster will be the rate at which toxins and harmful wastes are discharged from your body. This means that increasing the level of physical activity can, to some extent, mitigate the effects of an unhealthy diet. This does not mean, of course, that you can be careless about what you eat simply because you live a physically active life. However, it does mean that you must be more vigilant in working towards a healthy diet if the circumstances do not allow you an active lifestyle with a sufficient amount of physical activity. It is important to remember, however, that irregular, excessive physical exercise, relative to what your body can endure, imposes excessive burden on your body's waste removal function, as more toxic wastes are generated when calories (sugar) are burned (oxidized) at a greater rate during excessive physical exercise. Excessive irregular physical exercises create increased oxidative stress to the body's cells and can be counterproductive.

Step 4. Acquire the Taste of the New Modified Healthier Diet.

As you become used to the new modified healthier diet over time, you will find that you have acquired a taste for it and no longer crave the old diet. Once you have completely acquired the new taste, you will find the old unhealthy diet distasteful, uninviting, or even repelling.

Step 5. Make the New Modified Healthier Diet a Habit.

Make the new modified healthier diet a habit, until you are ready to progress to the next stage of an even healthier diet. After a while, you will find that you have acquired the taste for the new healthier diet and that it is impossible to go back to the diet of the earlier stage.

Step 6. Advance to the Next Stage of an Even Healthier Diet.

Once your new healthier diet has become habitual, you can now attempt to advance to the next stage of an even healthier diet by moving up the ladder of List B.

Step 7. Repeat Steps 3 through 6 until You Have Reached Your Final Goal.

Repeat Steps 3 through 6 until you are satisfied with a physical and mental fitness level that you feel great about. Ideally your final diet should consist primarily of List A items supplemented by items from the upper echelon of List B. But an acceptable healthy diet may contain some amounts of middle echelon List B items. In general, a marine life-based diet is preferable to the land based, reflecting the fact that life first started in the marine environment.

Having gone through the seven steps of achieving and maintaining a healthy, balanced diet, it is well worth remembering that an excessive calorie intake can speed up the aging process through increased oxidative stress resulting from the ramping up of your metabolic rate. It is also worth noting that it is much easier to restrain from overeating and excessive calorie intake through a primarily plant-based diet than through a primarily animal-based diet, and that oxidative stress is made worse by animal-based diets while it is offset by plant-based diets high in antioxidants. Scientific evidence is clear that low-calorie diets will help slow down the aging process. This is because low-calorie diets and associated low metabolic rates help minimize the harmful effects of oxidative stress.

B. Some Observations on Species Diets and their Longevity

It is interesting to note that there appears to be a strong positive correlation between the proportion of plant material in the diet and the life span of species. Among marine mammals, we find that bowhead whales and blue whales, whose main diet consists of krill and plankton, have an average life span of 110 years (blue whales) to over 200 years (bowhead whales), while killer whales, whose main diet is a variety of fish live, only 50 – 60 years. Among land mammals, Asian and African elephants, both of whom are herbivores, have average life spans of 78 and 60 years respectively. Grizzly bears, whose main diet consists of plants, fruits, and fish, on the other hand, live 47 years on average, while such carnivores as lions, bobcats, and tigers live only 20 – 30 years. Primates like chimpanzees and orangutans, whose diet is mainly plants and fruits, have an average life span of more than 55 years. Generally speaking, the ocean species live longer than the land species. Ocean quahogs (a member of the clam family) live more than 400 years, with a maximum 507 recorded. Interestingly enough, their diet consists entirely of marine algae and seaweeds. Other marine species with long life spans include rough eye rockfish (205 years), red sea urchin (200 years) and orange roughy (189 years). Lake sturgeon (fresh water fish) has an average life span of 152 years. A tortoise, whose main diet is grass and leafy vegetables, can live anywhere between 150 to 250 years.

Of course, these observations do not necessarily suggest a definitive positive correlation between the proportion of plant material in a human diet and human life expectancy, let alone causation of the latter by the former. Species diets evolve over very, very long periods of time. Nevertheless, it is probable that these observations may be more than just a coincidence.

Even more interesting and striking to note, however, is the apparent positive correlation between the proportion of plant material and fish in a diet and the life expectancy among human tribes. It is well known that the residents of Okinawa in Japan have the longest average life expectancy in the world and the highest centenarian ratio (number of those aged 100 years or more) of 68 per 100,000 inhabitants. It is less well known that the residents of Shimane prefecture, in the main island of Japan, enjoy an even higher centenarian ratio of 90. Compare these numbers to the centenarian ratio of 46 for Japan as a whole. Shimane prefecture, by virtue of being surrounded by sea to the north and mountains to the south, is somewhat isolated from industrialized mainstream Japan. Geography makes the diet of the residents of both Okinawa and Shimane largely vegetarian and marine-life based.

It is also interesting to note that the Caribbean island of Barbados has the next highest centenarian ratio of 30 and Sardinia the next highest at 13.5. Naturally the inhabitants of an island are likely to have a diet with a high proportion of fish and marine products. So it is not surprising to find high centenarian ratios for Barbados and Sardinia. However, the fact that Barbados and Sardinia lag significantly behind Shimane, Okinawa and even Japan as a whole in their centenarian ratios, although they are among the leaders in the world, can perhaps be explained by the fact that the diet of the Japanese is not only rich in fish and other marine-life based products but also contains plenty of land and sea vegetables and bean-based products such as tofu and bean paste. A proposition that it is the proportion of plant matter, including sea vegetables, in a diet rather than fish that is chiefly responsible for the longevity of the residents of Shimane and Okinawa is supported by another observation that the life expectancy of 50 - 60 years for the Inuit Eskimos is one of the lowest among the Canadian provinces. The diet of Inuit Eskimos consists mainly of flesh food, including fish and very little plant matter. Equally important, the residents of Shimane, Okinawa, Barbados, and Sardinia do not rely on automobiles as a means of transportation to the same extent that other peoples in the industrialized world do. It is also worth noting that the islanders in general breathe cleaner air and live more active and less stressful lives, aside from healthier diets and thereby better meet the requirements of the triad equilibrium than do inlanders.

Perhaps the most interesting and important observation one can make in this regard is the fact that the residents of Shimane and Okinawa not only enjoy long lives but healthy and active long lives. Most centenarians there manage to avoid such chronic age-related diseases as Alzheimer's, cardiovascular disease, and cancer. Furthermore, many centenarians in Japan have been found to enjoy active sex lives as well. The fact that a significant portion of the residents of Shimane and Okinawa can expect to live healthy and active lives well beyond 100 years, and that it is highly unlikely that the diets and the lifestyle of these centenarians precisely meet the requirements of an ideal triad equilibrium, suggest that a maximum healthy life expectancy for humans, associated with an ideal triad equilibrium, could be much higher than what these numbers currently imply. In my view, it would not be unreasonable to speculate a maximum human healthy life expectancy to be 10 – 20 percent higher than what it currently is for the residents of Shimane and Okinawa in Japan. I have used a value of 125 for the maximum human healthy life expectancy associated with the ideal triad equilibrium for an average woman in her early fifties in the subsequent illustration.

> "*Too much exercise can be harmful. ... Extremely intense, long-term cardiovascular exercise, as can be seen in athletes who train for multiple marathons, has been associated with scarring of the heart and heart rhythm abnormalities. ... Inappropriate exercise can do more harm than good, with the definition of "inappropriate" varying according to the individual. For many activities, especially running and cycling, there are significant injuries that occur with poorly regimented exercise schedules. Injuries from accidents also remain a major concern, whereas the effects of increased exposure to air pollution seem only a minor concern.*"
>
> ~ *Wikipedia*

C. Achieving And Maintaining Physical Fitness

We have stressed the importance of appropriate levels of physical exercise as a critical component of the triad of three essential requirements for a healthy body and mind. The appropriate level of physical exercise depends on one's age and the present state of one's physical fitness among other factors. While recognizing the critical importance of appropriate level of physical exercise for healthy body and mind, it should also be stressed that over-exercise is just as harmful to human body as under-exercise. One should start with the moderate level of exercise his/her body can take comfortably and gradually increase the level of vigour and the duration of exercise. In general, however, no matter how fit you are, it must be recognized that certain types of exercise are best avoided if you are advanced in age, say over 60. These include the types of exercise that require running or that put undue pressure on the joints such as ankles and knees, your back and neck, or that constantly rock the brain. Needless to say, a moderate level or amount of exercise of any kind is acceptable as long as it is within the reasonable limit set by one's fitness level. Generally speaking, if you are over 60, physical activities such as running (especially repetitious fast running and abrupt stopping), hiking mountains or steep hills with irregular terrain, and playing singles games of tennis or badminton should be avoided, unless you are sufficiently physically fit to absorb comfortably the shocks to your joints that these activities generate. Instead, less strenuous activities such as walking, bicycling, dancing, swimming, gentle rowing, playing golf, and yoga are recommended. Jogging on asphalt pavements is fine, as long as you wear appropriately designed running shoes, but jogging on concrete pavements is not recommended. Needless to say, as emphasized repeatedly in earlier pages, oxidative-stress-generating excessive irregular physical exercises are to be avoided. During exercise, oxygen consumption can increase by a factor of more than 10. This leads to a large increase in the production of oxygen radicals. Studies show that excessive and irregular exercise can contribute to oxidative stress, while moderate regular and steady exercise lowers the count of oxygen radicals.

It is good to remind ourselves of the analogy of the human body to an automobile. To maximize its useful life expectancy, an automobile must be well maintained (a healthy balanced diet) and driven actively but with moderation (physical activity with moderation). It should not be left idle (lack of exercise) for lengthy periods of time. Nor should it be driven excessively at excessive speeds (strenuous exercise) for extended periods of time. A car that has a high mileage (excessive physical activity) has a shorter remaining life expectancy. But a car driven around in the city most of the time (lack of physical exercise), even with low mileage, has a shorter life span. To be sure, there are fundamental differences between a machine and a human body. A machine is made up of inorganic materials whereas the human body is an organic mechanism capable of regenerating dying cells, within limits, given an appropriate diet, amount and type of physical exercise, and mindset. However, the undeniable fact that even an organic mechanism cannot regenerate dying cells indefinitely means that, in the final analysis, the human body is also a machine with a limited life span. Leaving it idle to collect dust and rust will shorten its life span. At the same time, abusing it with excessive and strenuous physical activity will also shorten its life expectancy.

Every species has its normal expected life span determined by its evolutionary history, which can be lengthened or shortened by proper or improper maintenance of the body and mind. It's not just the maintenance of the body but also of the mind that affects the expected life span, not just for humans but for other animals as well. It is well-known that dogs suffer emotionally to the detriment of their physical health when their beloved master suddenly dies. It may be conjectured that, given a proper diet and a harmonious state of mind, the expected healthy life expectancy of a species including that of humans displays a certain relationship to the level of regular and steady physical exercise, such as the one depicted in the following diagram.

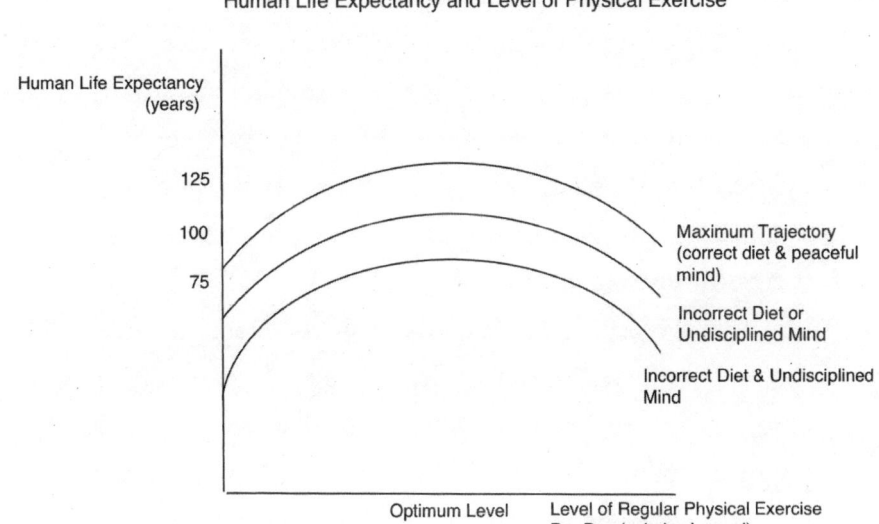

The diagram shows that there is an optimum level of regular daily exercise corresponding to the maximum expected healthy life span for humans, say 125 years for females, given a healthy, balanced diet and a peaceful and cheerful mind. As the level of regular daily exercise falls below the optimum level, the expected healthy life span drops below 125 years. The diagram also shows that the expected healthy life span drops below the maximum as the level of regular and steady daily exercise exceeds its optimum level. This is in part due to the excessive strain on the body. For example, vigorous physical activities, such as bodybuilding exercise and marathon running, if prolonged, may be too much even for a physically fit person to endure. In fact, the importance of avoiding sustained excessive physical exercise cannot be overemphasized. Sustained excessive physical exercise can cause premature aging through the oxidative stress effect. It can then be said that there are two opposing forces impinging on healthy life expectancy. One is a positive one: the physical fitness effect, or use-it-or-lose-it effect. The more actively parts of the body are used, the more physically fit the body becomes, other things being equal. The other is a negative one: wear-and-tear. Overly excessive use of the body will wear it out. If this is the case, there must be an optimum level of physical exercise that maximizes the physical fitness effect without triggering the wear-and-tear effect. [See the Mathematical Appendix at the end of the book.] The diagram also shows that the relationship between an expected healthy life expectancy and the level of regular and steady physical exercise will shift up or down as the quality of the diet and/or the level of mental fitness improves or deteriorates.

Quite apart from the wear-and-tear effect on the body, caused by excessive levels of physical activity, it is quite possible that there is also a built-in biological clock embedded in the system of every species, determined by its evolutionary history, and that excessive amount of physical activity may cause the biological clock to tick faster (in a manner analogous to running up of the mileage of an automobile) and cause a decrease in the remaining life span. It is quite possible that this biological clock sets the maximum human life expectancy associated with the optimum level of physical exercise, proper diet, and mental fitness. This biological-clock effect would be in addition to the wear-and-tear effect on the body. We must also recognize that, besides diet and physical and mental fitness, there may be other contributing factors, such as climate and other environmental factors, that can cause the relationship between the level of regular and steady exercise and the healthy life expectancy to shift.

Having recognized the fact that over-exercise is just as harmful to our body and mind as is under-exercise, it still is the case that in modern affluent industrial societies, in a vast majority of situations, it is under-exercise and lack of physical fitness that is the problem. Like a healthy, balanced diet, achieving physical fitness requires discipline. Allocating at least 30 to 40 minutes of your time every day to physical exercise should be a priority, whatever the type of exercise best suits your needs. If your work and other obligations do not allow even 30 minutes of daily exercise, try 15 minutes. Even 15 minutes is better than nothing if it can be kept regular and steady. Regularity and steadiness are two of the most important requirements. Regular and steady low-level exercise is more effective than irregular and intermittent vigorous exercise. Do not expect immediate results, particularly from low-level exercises. Achieving physical fitness requires a long-term commitment. Regular exercise should become a daily routine or habit, like eating and sleeping. It should be continued even during vacations and travel. When the routine is fully established and entrenched, it becomes an addiction, which is what one should aim for.

Admittedly most people will find it difficult to allocate even 30 minutes a day to physical exercise, particularly if your job requires leaving for work early in the morning and returning home late in the evening. But even in situations like this, you should be able to find time for something as critically important as improving your health and boosting your self-confidence. Most people should be able to squeeze 30 to 40 minutes for exercise in here and there during the course of a day. If this is not feasible for whatever reason, you may have to, as a last resort, sacrifice the amount of sleep you get by 30 minutes. This sacrifice, however, will be nothing compared to the huge payoff in return. In fact, it may be that the duration of sleep lost is more than compensated for by the increase in intensity of sleep, with the result that you haven't really lost the effective amount of sleep. Set the alarm 30 minutes earlier and do the exercise – say yoga, treadmill, or whatever suits you best – before you start the day. Can you find any compelling reason for not doing it? Too busy making money or chasing fame? Sacrificing one's health for the sake of making money or chasing fame has to be one of the most foolish things one can do to her/himself!

Probably it is young working parents, who must juggle endless tasks at home and at work plus minding their children's school work and extracurricular activities, who are confronted with the most challenging situations. For them, finding the time for regular and steady physical exercise may be all but impossible, or may be the last thing on their minds. For a single parent, the challenges can be even more daunting. I sympathize with them. My advice to them would be placing more emphasis on achieving and maintaining a healthy diet and a peaceful and cheerful mind than on physical exercise at this stage of their lives. Benefits of physical exercise increase with age. To young people, a properly balanced, healthy diet is more important for bodily health than is physical exercise. As one gets older, however, the appropriate level of physical exercise becomes increasingly important for maintaining a healthy body and mind within the triad. This does not mean, needless to say, that young people can neglect physical exercise all together. Young parents can play physically active games and sports with their children. Where there is a will, there is a way.

It appears that the benefits of triad equilibrium increase with age. The triad equilibrium is a matter of little significance for a child or a youth. As one gets older, however, the benefits of maintaining the triad equilibrium acquire greater and greater significance. This is because it becomes increasingly difficult to maintain a healthy body and mind as one's age increases. It also appears that the benefits of triad equilibrium increase with age at an accelerating rate rather than at a constant rate. This implies that people should pay increasingly closer attention to the triad equilibrium in their daily living as they get older.

> "Happiness is like a butterfly, which when pursued is just beyond your grasp, but which if you will sit down quietly may alight upon you."
> ~ Nathaniel Hawthorne

D. Disciplining Of The Mind

The benefits of keeping a peaceful and cheerful mind cannot be overemphasized. A disturbed mind causes oxidative stress and leads to ailments, both physical and mental. It is well established that a large portion of cancer incidence is attributable to a disturbed mind, which causes DNA damage through oxidative stress. Cancer initiation and promotion are associated with chromosomal defects and oncogene activation induced by free radicals. Studies have found that emotional stress increases free radical load on the body, as stress induces the release of hormones (such as adrenaline and cortisol), which mobilize the body in preparation for action – known as the fight or flight responses. This creates biochemical changes, which increase oxidative stress in the body. Oxidative stress also weakens the body's immune system. This makes the body vulnerable to attacks by disease-causing bacteria and viruses of all kinds. Emotional stress may be a result of such strong emotions as heartache, helplessness, frustration, and hatred, but other negative feelings such as greed, envy, jealousy, and prejudice can also contribute to it.

Emotional disturbances can be kept under control, and a peaceful and cheerful mind can be attained, through self-respect, respect for others, respect for nature, a positive attitude toward life, and occasional quiet moments. At the same time, a peaceful and cheerful mind bolsters self-respect, respect for others, and respect for nature, the key ingredients for the successful disciplining of the mind. Keeping a peaceful and cheerful mind makes it easier to maintain the discipline and self-respect required for maintaining a healthy, balanced diet and an appropriate level of physical exercise. Indeed, all elements of the triad reinforce each other in a virtuous circular chain. Working in reverse, should one link in the chain be weakened and left in disrepair for long, the chain will turn into a vicious circle destroying the mind and the body. Turning this around will require extraordinary effort, but once the virtuous circle has been restored, maintaining it will not be as hard. The trick is to make use of the momentum generated in the restorative process.

Some practical steps that are helpful in attaining a peaceful and cheerful mind suggest themselves. Immersing oneself in hobbies is an obvious example. Such hobbies might include drawing, painting, singing, playing musical instruments, writing poetry, dancing, favourite sports activities, going to concerts, movies, or shows, or just taking a walk. Just having quality time with family or friends can go a long way toward making your mind at peace and cheerful, perhaps even joyful. The list is endless. Meditation or yoga is a more systematic way of achieving a peaceful and cheerful mind. Have a positive attitude toward life. Be compassionate and generous to others and to yourself.

To most people, disciplining the mind may be the hardest of the three components of the triad. Do not burden yourself by setting too lofty a goal. You do not have to be a Saint or a Buddha to live peacefully and reach happiness. Whether through meditation or yoga or simply through deep breathing or looking up at the sky a few times a day, make it a habit. Do not expect quick results. The results from mind-disciplining efforts are gradual and may not be noticeable for years. However, remember this rule: The hardest thing to achieve is usually the most valuable thing to have: happiness! The two toughest internal enemies of happiness are greed and envy. If you can overcome greed and envy, you are almost there. Learn to be thankful for what you have. Your cup will be half full rather than half empty. Try to look at the bright side of everything, for everything has a bright side as well as a dark side. If you let go of greed and envy, look at the bright side of the world around you, and be genuinely thankful for what you have, you will truly be happy. Granted, the factors forced upon you externally, such as violence, trauma, betrayal, rejection, and isolation are difficult to deal with.

External factors such as these may be beyond your direct control, but to a large extent, you can deal with them by changing your attitude towards them, be it by plain acceptance or forgiveness. After all, things could have been worse. In fact, no matter what conditions you may be in, the chances are that there are many others on this planet who are worse off than you currently are. Remember that self-respect, respect for others, and respect for nature are the foundation for a peaceful and cheerful mind, which can be further enhanced through a positive attitude toward life and occasional quiet moments. Those with deep religious faith may find it easier to attain and maintain a peaceful and cheerful mind and perhaps even a joyful mind in their companionship with God, if they can maintain truly inclusive and accepting mind rather than being dogmatic and self-righteous.

Disciplining of the mind requires a disciplined effort. Discipline, however, must be distinguished from abstinence. Discipline is an act of voluntary will for the purpose of obtaining a goal. Abstinence, on the other hand, is a submission to externally imposed moral codes or religious edicts. An individual is free to accept or reject the discipline required for working towards a healthy life style. Abstinence is a suppression of natural instincts in one form or another. As such, it is unhealthy. Instincts are nature's way of signalling the body what basic needs must be satisfied for its survival. Suppressing or denying them is unhealthy. People are born with god-given natural instincts and inherent rights to pursue happiness through such secular pleasures as eating, sex, playing, and expression of thoughts and feelings through literature, arts and other creative activities. Natural instincts should not be suppressed and inherent rights should not be denied, although socially agreed moral codes or laws, which are designed for the betterment of the society, should be honoured. Discipline is a different matter. The primary reason for attempting to achieve and maintain a healthy life style is to make it possible to attain happiness. Discipline is only a means to this end.

What is happiness? Happiness is desire satisfied or fulfilled. Unhappiness is desire unsatisfied or unfulfilled. Desire makes you unhappy unless it is satisfied. The stronger is the desire, the greater will be the unhappiness unless it is satisfied. Stronger desire satisfied is greater happiness but stronger desire has less probability of being satisfied. Furthermore, stronger desires tend to beget even stronger desires upon being satisfied. This brings about a situation where you have to run faster and faster just to stay where you are. Moreover, the feeling of satisfaction one gets from a strong desire fulfilled does not last long, because even stronger desire awaits you at the doorstep of the one that has been fulfilled. Strong or excessive desire is greed and envy is its reflection. Moderate desire, on the other hand, has a better chance of being fulfilled than strong desire and the feeling of satisfaction one gets from moderate desires fulfilled tends to last longer. Hence, it may be said that the total accumulated feeling of satisfaction one gets from moderate desires fulfilled over a sufficiently long period time should be far greater than the total accumulated feeling of satisfaction from strong desires fulfilled over the same length of time. In fact, the chances are that a greedy or envious person will end up being quite unhappy due to the tendency for strong desires to become even stronger at successive stages over a sufficiently long period of time, because even stronger desires manifest themselves always one step ahead of the previously fulfilled ones. Happiness is within reach if your desires are kept at moderate levels. Happiness is a state of mind that one can control. Happiness is a feeling internally generated, not externally bestowed.

VIII. Closing Words

"Rivers know this: there is no hurry.
We shall get there some day."
~ A. A. Milne, *Winnie-the-Pooh*

THE THEORETICAL BASIS ON WHICH THE WELLNESS triad proposed here stands is the Darwinian theory of evolution, and the proposition of the wellness triad is strongly supported by accumulated scientific evidence. Species are naturally selected based on their ability to respond and adapt to their respective changing life environment. The human species is no exception. The life environment humans have had to respond and adapt to has undergone drastic, abrupt, and massive changes since the industrial revolution, on an unprecedented scale and to such an extent that these changes are having seriously damaging effects on human health. What is most alarming, however, is not that these changes have been taking place but that they are taking place at an ever-accelerating pace. This is nothing short of frightening. The damaging effects these changes inflict on human health occur on three different fronts: the foods we eat, the level of physical activity in which we engage, and the state of mind in which we find ourselves.

As for the foods we eat, we have been able to establish the following general principles based on careful analysis and examination of the accumulated scientific evidence within the framework of the Darwinian theory of evolution:

- The greater (smaller) is the evolutionary (genetic) distance of a food source from the human species, the more (less) beneficial to human health it is;

- the less is the degree of human intervention in growing or raising a food, the healthier it is;

- the less refined or processed is a food, the healthier it is; and

- the less intensively cooked is a food, the healthier it is.

Of these, the first principle on the relationship between a food source's evolutionary distance from the human species and its health benefits to humans is a new discovery, and it is of paramount importance of the four. The entire Chapter V was devoted to the examination and analysis of the accumulated scientific evidence supporting these principles. The evidence has been found to be strongly consistent with the Darwinian theory of evolution. In fact, the evidence appears to be rock solid. The unfortunate reality is that, despite such clear and strong evidence, the principles stated above are not wholeheartedly embraced and certainly not widely practised by the community of health professionals, much less by the general public. No doubt parts of these principles are accepted by some as common sense but certainly not whole-heartedly embraced and practised in their daily lives – if the current average state of health of the adult population in the industrialized world is any indication, as pointed out by the World Health Organization. I attribute this to the tendency of not seeing the forest for the trees on the part of the community of health professionals and the scientific community in general, which prevents them from seeing the world from a broader historical perspective. This unfortunate reality is the reason for my writing this book. In this book, these principles have been used to develop the guidelines for establishing a healthy, balanced diet. The six intermediate steps (seven including the final step) for attaining and maintaining the goal of healthy, balanced diet have been suggested and explained.

As for the level of physical activity we engage in, we have seen that an appropriate level of physical activity varies from individual to individual depending on such factors as individual's age, sex, and existing fitness level. Further, given the diet and mental/emotional state, we have seen that there exists a quadratic relationship between the amount of physical exercise and the maximum healthy life expectancy of an individual. That is, healthy life expectancy of an individual is positively related to the amount of steady and regular physical activity he or she engages in, only up to a point, beyond which it becomes an inverse relationship. In other words, not only is under-exercise unhealthy but so is over-exercise. There is an optimum level of regular and steady exercise for an individual associated with the maximum healthy life expectancy, given their diet, state of mind, and other environmental factors. An exercise level higher than the optimum is just as unhealthy as one that is lower than this. Often neglected is the fact that physical activity must be regular and steady for it to have a maximum beneficial effect. In fact, it has been found that highly irregular excessive physical exercise is harmful to the body because of the oxidative stress it generates. In any case, certain types of strenuous exercise are best to be avoided by the individuals who are advanced in age, although the critical importance of moderate, regular, and steady exercise (particularly for individuals of advanced age) cannot be overemphasized.

The third element of the triad, that is, maintaining peaceful and cheerful mind, is just as important as the other two for the overall health of the body and mind. Maintaining peaceful and cheerful mind on a continuous basis is not something that is easily achieved. The trick here is not to aim too high but to be patient and steady with a long term goal in mind. Learn to be thankful for what you have. You will find that you have so much to be thankful for. Greed and envy are two of the worst enemies of a peaceful and cheerful mind. Self-respect, respect for others, and respect for the environment are the minimum requirements for achieving and maintaining a peaceful and cheerful mind.

When the three requirements are fully met, each of the three components of the triad supports each other in a state of stable equilibrium. This may be referred to as the wellness-triad equilibrium. Once the equilibrium has been achieved, it does not easily unravel and has a tendency to persist. This is because each of the components supports the other two. Even if one of the components suffers due to unavoidable external shock such as unforeseen accidents, death in the family and the like, the other two strong components will make it easier for this component to recover quickly. However, building the triad equilibrium from the scratch requires much greater effort. Once it has been achieved, it is much easier to maintain. It is to be recognized that the benefits of the triad equilibrium increase with age. Not only do they increase with age but they increase at an accelerating rate as one gets older. This is easy to see. It is much easier for an 18-year old youth to stay reasonably healthy than for a 65-year old senior even when their diets, exercise levels and states of mind deviate temporarily from the ideal state for some reason, perhaps some external factor beyond their control. Although it is undoubtedly true that health of a youth will suffer from poor diet, inactive lifestyle and emotional trauma to some extent, the extent to which health of an elderly person will suffer from similar shocks to the triad equilibrium is bound to be much greater and the speed of recovery much slower. In fact, for an elderly person, a full recovery may be impossible under certain circumstances or extremely slow even when possible once the triad equilibrium has been seriously damaged by a grave failure of even one component of the three. This is the reason why, as one gets older, s/he needs to pay an increasingly closer attention to the requirements of the wellness-triad equilibrium.

In closing, two things deserve to be emphasized. First, do not expect quick results. Truly valuable things in life are not easily obtained, but they are worth the effort. You should be prepared to work for them. You will be rewarded in proportion to the amount of effort you put in. Second, the effort you must make does not have to be a struggle. Frequently on a journey, what matters most is not necessarily the destination itself but how you reach that destination. Try to savour the progress you make. Having this attitude will make your journey more enjoyable. Try to have fun doing it. Even if you do not reach the final destination that you have set for yourself, all is not lost as long as progress is being made and you are having fun doing it.

Most of all, enjoy what you do for a living. Have fun at work but also put your best effort into it. Do not sacrifice fun and health for the sake of a career or financial success. Money cannot buy health or happiness. If you ruin your health for the sake of building a financial fortune or a successful career, what good is it? Enjoying what you do for a living and doing your best at work will probably give you the best chance for a successful career. Putting the seven principles for healthy living into practise should also be fun. You should do it with pleasure and a feeling of excitement. Life should be fun, not a struggle. This means living in harmony with nature, not working against it!

Through the ages, kings and emperors have sought in vain for a miracle potion for extending their lives (elixir of life). As always, the truth lies right before your eyes and it is tantalizingly plain and simple. Now you have it. The hard part is making up your mind to put it into practise. As Helen Keller said, ideas without action are worthless. Like everything, however, once you put your mind to it, it is not all that hard after all.

A Mathematical Appendix

[This section is mainly for the benefit of those readers who are mathematically inclined and may be skipped by general readers without loss of critically important contents.]

THE APPROPRIATE LEVEL OF PHYSICAL EXERCISE IS one of the three pillars of good health for the body and the mind. What is the appropriate level of physical exercise? It is difficult to pin down quantitatively, although it is safe to say that whatever level of exercise makes you feel great about your body and mind must be the right or ideal level. Too little or too much exercise, relative to the ideal level, is equally sub-optimal in the sense that it prevents your body and mind from achieving the maximum potential. The maximum potential can be defined as the highest attainable, healthy life expectancy.

There are two conflicting effects of physical exercise that impinge on a healthy life expectancy. The first is a positive one: increasing healthy life expectancy through the physical fitness effect or use-it-or-lose-it effect. The second is a negative one: the wear-and-tear effect or oxidative-stress effect. The two opposing effects may be captured by a quadratic equation such as:

$$y = -ax^2 + bx + c$$

where y represents a healthy life expectancy measured in years, x represents the level of regular and steady daily physical exercise measured by the number of calories burned per day expressed as a ratio relative to a baseline sedentary level, and a, b, and c are positive constants. The first term of the equation captures the wear-and-tear effect and the second term the physical fitness effect. The ideal level of physical exercise is that level which maximizes a healthy life expectancy, i.e., x= (1/2)(b/a). [Solve dy/dx = -2ax + b = 0 for x.] For a quadratic equation, say, y = -60x² + 230x - 95, the ideal solution for x is 1.92, i.e., 92 percent over the average number of calories burned per day associated with a sedentary life style for an average woman in her early fifties, given a healthy, balanced diet and harmonious state of mind. The average number of calories burned per day by a woman with a sedentary life style in her early fifties is about 1,600. This means that the optimum number of calories to be burned per day for an average woman in her early fifties is approximately 3,072. The maximum healthy life expectancy associated with this level of regular and steady daily exercise, given a healthy, balanced diet and a harmonious state of mind, is 125.4 years.

Thus, in this illustration, a maximum healthy life expectancy of 125.4 years is achieved at the regular and steady daily exercise level corresponding to 92 percent above the average number of calories burned per day by an average woman with a sedentary life style in her early fifties. Up to this level, the physical fitness effect dominates the wear-and-tear effect, while above this level the latter effect dominates the former. In this illustration, as the regular and steady daily exercise level increases from zero percent ($x = 1.0$) to 50 percent ($x = 1.5$) above the sedentary level, the healthy life expectancy rises from 75 years to 115 years. Having reached the maximum healthy life expectancy of 125.4 years associated with 92 percent ($x = 1.92$) above the sedentary level of exercise, however, further increase in the exercise level results in a decrease in healthy life expectancy. Thus, as the regular and steady daily exercise level increases from 150 percent ($x = 2.5$) to 190 percent ($x = 2.9$) above the sedentary level, for example, the healthy life expectancy falls from 105 years to 67.4 years. This relationship, of course, holds for an ideal diet combined with mental fitness. The relationship can be expected to shift down as the diet and/or the mental fitness level fall(s) short of the ideal level(s). Environmental factors such as climate would also cause the relationship to shift.

It must also be recognized that there may be a biological-clock effect of the excessive physical exercise, quite apart from its wear-and-tear effect, that has not been captured by this equation. The biological-clock effect is the effect on the life expectancy of causing the biological clock to tick faster by speeding up the rate of metabolism through excessive exercise. The biological clock of each species is assumed to have been set genetically by the evolutionary history of the species. The biological-clock effect would accentuate the wear-and-tear effect of the excessive physical exercise over the optimal level.

In the illustration represented by the above equation, up to 125.4 years of maximum healthy life expectancy for an average woman in early fifties, the physical fitness effect of regular and steady physical exercise dominates its wear-and-tear effect. Beyond that point, however, the latter effect dominates the former. These numbers are mainly for illustrative purposes but may not be utterly unreasonable considering the fact that the current maximum healthy life expectancy for the residents of Shimane and Okinawa in Japan exceeds 100 years by a significant margin and that it is highly unlikely that those centenarians of Shimane and Okinawa have necessarily achieved the triad equilibrium for a maximum healthy life expectancy.

Index

acid-forming 45-7, 49, 70, 101
acidosis 45, 47, 94
adipose tissue 38
adrenaline 52, 58, 119
alkaline-forming 46, 70, 97
amoeba 5
amylopectin 48
amylose 48
antioxidant 40-1, 43, 51-2, 57, 70, 78-9, 83, 97
archaea 5, 63
artery wall 32-3, 70
atherosclerosis 42, 98

bacteria 5, 29, 48, 63-4, 119
Barbados 107-8
Bekoff, Marc 23
Bentham, Jeremy 84
beta-carotene 40
biological clock effect 81, 115, 136
biological extinction 9
biosphere 5
bipedalism 13
blood pH 32, 41, 44-5, 49, 70, 94

bromine 94, 101
Buddha 120
buffering system 44-5, 47, 49, 70, 94

calcium hydroxide 48
calcium phosphate 45-7
cannibalism 15, 69
cardiovascular disease 35, 42
cell cycle 41
cell membrane 32-3, 37-8, 40, 42, 58, 63, 70, 78
cellular respiration 39, 51, 64
centenarian ratio 107-8, 136
Cheung, Lilian 83
chimpanzee 1, 14, 23, 106
cholesterol, blood 32-5, 49-50, 62
cholesterol, dietary 33-5, 68
cholesterol (HDL) 34-6, 70
cholesterol (LDL) 34-6, 62, 68, 70
chloroplast 64
common ancestor 1, 3, 5, 14
constrained optimization 4, 27-8
cortisol 52, 58, 119

Dalai Lama 82
Darwin, Charles xvii, 2, 6, 11, 18, 125-7
Dawkins, Richard 6, 28, 31, 63
deoxyribonucleic acid (DNA) 40-2, 58, 63-4, 70, 78, 118
diabetes, type 1 38
diabetes, type 2 38-9, 51-2
dietary fibre 47, 65, 98
differential equation 27
dinosaur 9, 29
diverticulitis 98
divine intention 23
Dominy, Nathaniel 13-4, 71

economic problem 4, 27
Einstein, Albert 2
electrolyte equilibrium 100
electromagnetic force 2
elixir of life 131
emergence of life 4
environmental shock 8, 31, 50, 62, 82
eukaryotic cell 5, 63-64
evolution (theory of) 3, 6, 10, 69, 125-7
evolutionary adaptation xvi, 9-10, 12, 15-6, 19, 47, 59, 73, 77, 87
evolutionary distance 14-6, 35-6, 39, 43, 46, 49, 68-9, 71, 93-5, 126
evolutionary cousin 14, 69
evolutionary tree 15
external shock xvi, 8-9, 11-2, 73

fat, hydrogenated 34, 42, 70
fat, saturated 33-6, 39, 68, 70
fat, trans 33-4
fat, unsaturated 34-5, 68, 70
fat, mono-unsaturated 34
fat, poly-unsaturated 34, 68
fatty acid, long chain 36
fatty acid, medium chain 36
fight and flight response 52, 58, 119
flavonoid 43
free fatty acid 38, 51
free radical 39-41, 43, 51-2, 70, 78-9, 83, 119
fundamental forces (of nature) 1-4, 27-8

G1 (growth) phase 41
genetic ability xvii-iii, 8
genetic distance 14, 49, 68, 126
genetic mutation 28, 41
glucagon 37
glucose 37-8, 52, 98
gravitational force 2

happiness 24-5, 84, 86, 121-3
Hawthorne, Nathaniel 118
healthy balanced diet 33, 55, 61, 65, 87-91, 94-5, 102, 105, 112-3, 119, 127, 134-5
healthy life expectancy 109, 115, 128, 133-6
heart disease 32, 43, 50, 98
homeostasis 12, 37, 49
human chauvinist 22

human diet evolution 13
human physiology xvii, 7, 15, 29,
    49-50, 55, 65
hydrogenated vegetable oil 34

ideal body weight 56, 85-86
immune system 11-2, 42, 51-2,
    56, 58, 119
industrial revolution 16, 125
insulin receptor 37-8
insulin resistance 32, 37-8, 49,
    51, 62
insulin spike 48-9, 98
intermediate target diet 90,
    93-4, 101-3
intestinal bacteria 48
Inuit Eskimo 108

Keller, Helen 87, 131
kidney stone 46

life environment xvi, 7-9
life expectancy (healthy) 16-7,
    26-7, 81, 107, 109, 112-5, 128,
    133, 135-6
lipoprotein, high density
    (HDL) 33
lipoprotein, low density (LDL)
    33, 42
Lindlahr, Victor 75
love 84-5
lysozyme 12

marginal benefit 28
marginal cost 28
metabolic process 42, 64, 73

metabolism, anaerobic 41
metabolism, aerobic 40-1
Metropolitan Toronto Zoo 23
Milne, A. A. 125
mindful living 83
missing link 1
mitochondrion(a) 64

natural selection xvii, 6,
    10-1, 125

obesity epidemic xv
Okinawa 107-9, 136
origin of species 3
oxidative stress 32, 36, 39, 41-4,
    47, 49, 51, 58, 62, 70, 78-9,
    81, 83, 104-5, 111, 114, 118-9,
    128, 134
oxidative phosphorylation 39
oxygen radical 39-40, 111

package of natural laws xvii
pancreas 37-8
pathogen 12, 40
phosphorus-calcium balance 47
photosynthesis 5, 64, 69
physiological adaptation 14, 16
premature human mortality xv
prokaryotic cell 5, 63

quadratic relationship 128, 134

ribonucleic acid (RNA) 5,
    42, 63-4
ribosome 64
Ridley, Matt 1

Sardinia 107-8
scurvy 15
self-defense mechanism 11-2, 40,
    73, 78
self-sustaining equilibrium 37
seven principles (for healthy
    living) xvii-iii, 8, 55-6, 87, 131
Shimane 107-9, 136
Stevenson, Robert Louis 60
stroke 32, 33, 35-6, 43, 50, 98
strong nuclear force 2
survival of the fittest xvii, 6

Thich Nhat Hanh 83, 101
triad (wellness) xvii-iii, 62, 88-9,
    110, 117, 119, 125, 128-9
triad (wellness) equilibrium xviii,
    53, 61-2, 108-9, 118, 129-
    130, 136

virus 29, 119

Wallace, Alfred Russell 2
weak nuclear force 2
Wikipedia 110
Winnie-the-Pooh 125
World Health Organization
    xv, 127

xenobiotics 11-2

Printed in Canada